1,001 WAYS TO USE ESSENTIAL OILS

1,001 WAYS TO USE ESSENTIAL OILS

by

Beth Jones

First published November 2014

ISBN-13: 978-1503193246

ISBN-10: 1503193241

Table of Contents

1

Essential Oils

What are Essential Oils?

Essential oils are aromatic, highly concentrated plant extracts derived directly from the bark, petals, rinds, roots, resins, or seeds of the plant itself. Throughout history, these oils have been used in a variety of different ways to improve health and happiness. Essential oils were used medicinally as far back as Ancient Greece, being used in household items and spiritual worship. The Ancient Egyptians used them in the mummification process and in sacred ceremonies, while people were using such plants for medicinal and religious purposes in many areas of the Far East, notably India and China. Certain essential oils like tea tree oil were often used to combat illness and disease before the development of modern antibiotics. It is reported that perfumers and spice merchants in the Middle Ages, who knew the medicinal properties of essential oils, were able to avoid becoming infected with the Plague by using the oils. During WWI and WWII medicines like antibiotics were in short supply on the battlefields of Europe so medics and field doctors would use essential oils like lavender to treat burns and guard against infection and sepsis.

Essential oils are truly complex chemical compounds, each containing many different components, which act on the body in a variety of different ways. In order to obtain the essential oil from a specific part of a plant, several different extraction methods are used including, steam distillation, expression, solvent extraction, and enfleurage. While steam distillation is the most popular method, all are equally as important.

The harvesting of the plants used to create essential oils is a delicate and complex process. Farmers will often wait until certain times of the day or night to gather the plants, knowing that the oils will be at their highest quality. Once this is done, the plants are then taken to the manufacturing area, which is often in very close proximity to the fields in order to preserve the goodness of the plant. It is here that the essential oils are meticulously extracted using one of the methods mentioned above.

Essential oils, or essences as they are also known, are 100% natural, containing no contaminants, preservatives, or addictives. They are often called the 'life force' of the plant as they contain its vital energy. It is this energy that can have such a potent effect on the human mind and body.

How Do Essential Oils Work?

Essential oils help to balance the body's systems, fight against fungal and viral infections, strengthen and support the immune system, reduce inflammation, fight the signs of aging, provide relief from pain, improve digestion, relieve respiratory tract disorders, stimulate circulation, calm the nervous system, and so much more.

These magical oils carry out these therapeutic actions in 3 ways;

◆Inhalation
◆Skin Absorption
◆Ingestion

Inhalation

When you inhale the scent of an essential oil, its aromatic molecules infuse the air around you and as you inhale, these fine molecules travel up through the nose into the olfactory receptors – structures within the nasal airways which process smells. Once the receptors have processed the smell, a message is relayed to the limbic system of the brain. This is the area of the brain where emotions are controlled. The hypothalamus, the area of the brain that controls hormones, is also stimulated.

Scent has a very powerful effect on emotions and on the brain. Certain smells can unconsciously trigger emotions and repressed memories, and activate the production of certain hormones. The limbic system also influences the nervous system and as a result, essential oils can either stimulate or calm physiological and psychological responses in the body. The effect on the brain is almost immediate, which makes essential oils a safe and quick treatment for various problems.

When you inhale essential oils, the molecules also enter the respiratory system, where they can have a positive influence on coughing, bronchitis, asthma, colds & flu, and sinusitis. These molecules are also passed directly into the bloodstream where they are carried to certain cells in the body to trigger healing.

Skin Absorption

The tiny molecules contained within essential oils are effectively absorbed by the skin. Here, these molecules promote cell regeneration, reduce inflamed or irritated skin, improve the elasticity of skin, and reduce the formation of wrinkles. They are also transported to muscles and organs in the body by the bloodstream, and can therefore help to ease muscle aches and pains, alleviate spasms in muscles and intestines, stimulate digestion, and help to fight various fungal, viral, and bacterial infections.

The phenols and monoterpenes contained within essential oils are two ingredients that are important for keeping cells healthy. Phenols, when absorbed into the skin, help to clean out the receptor area of cells so that they can function more effectively and fight off free radicals and toxins. Monoterpenes also prevent the build up of toxins in the cells and have the amazing ability to restore DNA in an otherwise unhealthy cell. Once the DNA is reversed and the cells are healthy, they can fight off disease, therefore helping to maintain balance in the body.

Ingestion

When ingested, essential oils are absorbed directly into the bloodstream through the digestive system. Some essential oils are used in flavorings, mouth rinses, and toothpaste such as peppermint, nutmeg, or spearmint. For the most part, it is not recommended to ingest essential oils unless otherwise advised by a medical practitioner.

2

Storage & Safety of Essential Oils

Choosing & Storing Essential Oils

Choosing the finest pure essential oils is an extremely important factor in determining how effective the aromatherapy blend or treatment will be, and with the large selection of essential oils available on the market along with a growing number of suppliers, this task can be a daunting one. Before choosing an essential oil brand, it is important to carry out an adequate amount of research first, taking into account the following considerations;

◆ Purity ◆ Quality ◆ Price ◆ Storage

Purity
Choose oils that are 100% essential oils, ones that are not synthetics, dilutions or adulterations. Avoid terms such as "nature-identical", "fragrance oil" or "perfume oil" as these types of oils will often have chemical or artificial ingredients added to them. Additives and adulteration (meaning adjusting or altering the oil in some way) have the potential to be harmful to the body and they also create weak, ineffective results in aromatherapy.

Quality
The quality of an essential oil is determined by a number of factors including;

◆ The plant species
◆ The quality of the soil
◆ The weather conditions/temperature
◆ Where the plants are grown – indoors/outdoors
◆ The extraction method used

The actual bottle of essential oil will not provide this information so this is where proper research comes into play. A reputable company should monitor the production of their oils from start to finish, and provide the general public with information on how they carry out this process. Always research the company's website and any literature they provide.

Price

The price of essential oil varies enormously and depends on how difficult or easy it is to extract the oil from the plant. For example, 2 million rose petals are needed to make just 1 ounce of Rose oil, making it one of the most expensive essential oils on the market. Alternatively it takes approximately 30kg of eucalyptus leaves to make 1 liter of Eucalyptus oil, making it one of the lesser expensive oils. When choosing, make sure the oils are not unusually cheap, especially the more expensive ones like Rose, Melissa, Neroli or Jasmine. This could mean they may not be pure or of good quality. It is a good idea to compare different brands to get an overall idea of how much your chosen essential oils should cost.

Storage

Essential oils are precious and expensive. It is therefore vital that they are stored correctly to ensure both their longevity and effectiveness. When you are purchasing oils or creating a blend at home, the following factors should be adhered to, to ensure you get the most from you oils;

> Make sure they are contained within dark amber or cobalt blue bottles. Sunlight can have a detrimental effect on the chemistry of essential oils causing them to deteriorate rapidly and lose their therapeutic benefits. Dark colored glass bottles offer protection from the sun's harmful ultra violet rays.

> Ensure the bottles are tightly sealed. Any prolonged contact with the air will cause essential oils to lose their composition and evaporate.

> Keep essential oils stored in a cool, dry place. Do not store them in an area where they will be subject to extreme changes in temperature. The heat will evaporate the oil whereas the cold will cause it to lose its composition.

> When purchasing essential or carrier oils, never buy oils that have dust on the cap or bottle. This is a sure sign that they have been sitting there for some time. Don't be afraid to ask the retailer when the oils arrived into the shop.

> Avoid aluminum or plastic bottles as the molecular structure of the oil will be affected.

Most essential oils have a shelf life of at least 2 years, particularly ones that have gone through steam distillation. There are some exceptions to this however, so make sure you do some research first (Tea Tree oil normally lasts for approximately 12 to 18 months).

Citrus oils like Lemon, Orange, Bergamot, Mandarin or Neroli have the shortest shelf life of around 9 to 12 months.

It is important to note that carrier oils should be treated with as much careful consideration. They will go rancid very quickly if not stored properly. Most carrier oils have a shelf life of up to 2 years, with the exception of borage oil and flaxseed oil – these are very delicate and have a shelf life of about 6 months. Coconut and jojoba oils last for about 4 years and are often added to other carrier oils to extend the shelf life of a blend.

Treating them with the love and attention they deserve will ensure they last longer, providing you with outstanding therapeutic benefits.

Use the following checklist as a guide when purchasing your essential oils:

Is the Latin name of the plant provided? This will ensure you are getting the correct variation of a particular oil, for example, there are several varieties of eucalyptus.
Where is the oil from? Sometimes quality can vary between countries.
What is the purity of the oil? It should be 100% essential oil. Avoid terms like "nature-identical", "fragrance oil" and "perfume oil".
Is the essential oil stored in a dark amber or cobalt blue glass container?
Are the bottles sealed tightly? If the seals have been broken, the oil could be compromised so avoid.
Where are the oils stored? Are they away from heaters or radiators? Are they away from direct sunlight?
How long has the oil been in stock?
How has the essential oil been extracted? This will give you an indication as to its shelf life.
Are the prices comparable to other brands? If they are unusually cheap, they could be dilutions so be careful.
Are the more expensive oils like Rose or Jasmine priced the same as say, Lemongrass or Rosemary? If so, they are more than likely diluted.

The Safety of Essential Oils

Used correctly, essential oils are very safe and can be used effectively to treat a number of specific conditions such as dry skin or insomnia. There is however, a possibility that oils used in the wrong dilutions or the overuse of any particular oil, may cause irritation and produce adverse effects. To prevent this from happening, there are several safety guidelines that should be followed, ensuring that you get the best from your blend.

❖ Allergy testing – before using an essential oil for the first time, particularly if you have sensitive skin or suffer from allergies, it is important you carry out a patch test on a small area of skin. To do this;

1. Blend 5ml of your chosen carrier oil along with 4 drops of essential oil, and apply to a small section on the inside of your elbow.
2. Apply a plaster or bandage over the area and leave for 24 hours.
3. If you encounter any symptoms such as itching, redness, inflammation, stinging or rash, remove the essential oil with cool, clean water.
4. If no irritation occurs after the 24 hour period, then you know it is safe to use.

Some carrier oils may contain traces of nut so it is imperative to avoid these oils if you suffer from nut allergies. Peanut and Hazelnut oils are obvious examples but all carrier oils should be checked before use.

❖ Skin irritants – while you may not have experienced any adverse reactions to the patch test, there are certain essential oils that can be irritating to the skin and should therefore be used with care. These include; *Basil, Benzoin, Black pepper, Cinnamon, Clove, Ginger, Lemon, Lemongrass, Melissa, Orange, Oregano, Peppermint, Pine, Thyme, Tea tree.*

❖ Medication – using essential oils while taking medication is not recommended as some oils can interfere with certain prescription medication. Always consult your doctor before using any oil.

❖ Photosensitivity – certain essential oils (mainly citrus oils) contain constituents that absorb sunlight/UV rays, increasing the effect sun can have on the skin. Using these oils before going out into the sun or using the sun bed can increase your chances of hyper pigmentation, sunburn, blisters or rash. The following oils should be avoided prior to UV exposure; *Bergamot, Lemon, Lemongrass, Mandarin, Orange, Lime, Grapefruit.*

- ❖ Avoid contact with the eyes. If any essential oil enters the eyes, rinse out immediately with plenty of cold water.
- ❖ Never use essential oils during the 1st trimester of pregnancy. For the remainder of the term, consult with your doctor before using any essential oils as most are not recommended.

- ❖ Never ingest essential oils unless it clearly states the nutritional content and instructions for use on the label.

- ❖ Essential oils should never be used on open cuts or wounds.

- ❖ With the vast number of essential oils available, there are some which should be completely avoided due to their toxicity. The following is a list of toxic oils which should never be used, under any circumstances;

Aniseed	Pennyroyal
Arnica	Rue
Bitter Almond	Sage
Boldo	Sassafras
Broom	Savin
Buchu	Savory
Calamus	Tansy
Camphor	Thuja
Cassia	Tonka
Horseradish	Wintergreen
Jaborandi	Wormseed
Mugwort	Wormwood

3
How to Use
Essential Oils

Essential oils are highly concentrated and should not be applied to the skin in their pure undiluted form (lavender and tea tree are exceptions to this rule). It is important to blend the essential oil in a carrier oil before use. Examples of excellent carrier oils include coconut, olive, apricot kernel, almond, grapeseed, evening primrose, jojoba, avocado, and wheatgerm.

Essential oils need to be diluted at a ratio of .5 to 3%, depending on the person's skin, the strength and/or toxicity of the oil, the condition it is being used for, and the area to be treated. The following methods are the most common ways essential oils can be incorporated into everyday living.

In the Bath
This is perhaps the most effective and easiest way to use essential oils. Simply dilute a number of drops in 1 tablespoon of carrier oil, and add to a bath. Always run the bath first before adding the oils. Depending on the oil, you can use anywhere between 2 and 8 drops of essential oil to 1 tablespoon of carrier oil. Never exceed 10 drops.

This is a great way to reduce anxiety and stress, ease muscular aches and pains, promote a good night's sleep, ease cystitis and hemorrhoids, alleviate PMS, and reduce restlessness.

Inhalation
To inhale the oils, you can either place a couple of drops on a tissue, or add several drops to a steam inhalation. The steam inhalation is very effective when trying to relieve coughing, colds, bronchitis, and congestion. Oily skin and open pores can also be treated successfully using this method. If you need a little energy boost, 2 drops of a stimulating oil on a tissue can work wonders.

Vaporizer/Diffuser
Whether you want to promote a peaceful night's sleep, ease breathing, promote positive feelings, increase focus and concentration, or repel annoying insects, vaporizing essential

oils can be quick and effective. Always place a tablespoon of water at the top of the burner, along with your chosen oils.

Compress

A compress is a piece of material, typically a muslin cloth or a soft face cloth, that is soaked in either hot or cold water, and applied directly to a specific part of the body. A cold compress is traditionally used to treat localized swelling, joint sprains, headaches and insect bites. Meanwhile, a hot compress is more suitable for muscular aches and pains, earache, toothache and menstrual cramps. Simply place 2-3 drops of your chosen oil on the compress. and place over the area of concern.

Massage

With the wide array of therapeutic properties offered by essential oils, their popularity in massage comes as no surprise. Massage in its own right offers many fantastic benefits to both our body and mind, but when you throw essential oils into the mix, these benefits are dramatically enhanced. A massage can take the form of a facial, full body, or localized massage. It can alleviate insomnia, reduce stress and tension, ease muscle soreness, reduce inflammation, improve circulation, and promote the elimination of toxins and wastes from the body. The essential oils should always be diluted in a carrier oil, with no more than 12 drops of oil being used for a full body massage.

Foot Bath

This is a great way to soothe tired, aching feet, fight athlete's foot, reduce swelling, and stimulate circulation. Dilute drops of your chosen oil in carrier oil, and add to the foot bath.

Neat Application

Lavender is an excellent oil to use on boils, cold sores, abrasions, bites, stings, spots, warts, and verrucae. Simply apply 1 neat drop of oil onto the problem area. Tea tree oil can also be used but caution must be taken as it can cause sensitivity and skin irritation.

4

Therapeutic Actions of Essential Oils

Each essential oil has individual properties and characteristics of its own. While some possess similar attributes, others can be very different. It is therefore important to understand the potential therapeutic actions of each essential oil so you can choose the right one for you. If, for example, you suffered from insomnia, you would not choose peppermint oil as it is very stimulating in nature and would subsequently affect a peaceful night's sleep.

A reputable essential oil company will always list the therapeutic actions of their oils so you can clearly match an oil to your specific needs. Below is a list of common terminology used to describe various properties contained within essential oils;

Analgesic – reduces the sensation of pain. A substance that contains an analgesic acts as a pain killer.

Anti-allergic – prevents or reduces allergic reactions.

Anticatarrhal – helps to remove excess mucus from the body.

Antidepressant – helps lift the symptoms of depression such as low moods and sadness; instils feeling on happiness, optimism and hope.

Anti-inflammatory – reduces inflammation and swelling.

Antimicrobial – a general term that describes an oil that possesses antibacterial, antifungal and antiviral properties. An antimicrobial kills microorganisms or inhibits their growth.

Antipruritic – helps to relieve or prevent itching.

Antiseptic – a property that is capable of preventing infection by inhibiting the growth of microorganisms.

Antispasmodic – helps to reduce or prevent spasms, contractions or convulsions.

Antiviral – helps to destroy a viral infection, it can also prevent one from occurring.

Aphrodisiac – heightens sexual desire.

Astringent – a substance that causes the contraction or shrinking of body tissues, and helps to dry up secretions.

Antitussive – a cough suppressant; relieves coughing.

Bactericidal – kills bacterial growth or prevents bacteria from growing.

Balancing – creates balance in the emotions to bring about a homeostatic effect on the body.

Calming – produces a calming, relaxing effect on either the body, mind or both.

Carminative – helps to prevent or relieve flatulence; gas in the gastrointestinal tract.

Cholagogue – promotes the discharge of bile from the gall bladder and ducts.

Cicatrisant – an agent that heals a wound by the formation of scar tissue.

Cooling – cools an area of the body; lowers temperature.

Cytophylactic – stimulates the regeneration of new cells; preserving the health of the skin and tissues.

Deodorant – removes or covers up body odor or unpleasant smells.

Depurative – cleanses and removes impurities and toxins from the blood; purifies the blood.

Diaphoretic – induces perspiration.

Diuretic – a substance that increases the production of urine in the kidneys.

Emmenagogue – helps to provoke menstruation when periods are irregular or missing.

Emollient – softens or soothes the skin.

Expectorant – promotes the removal of mucus from the lungs, bronchi, and trachea.

Febrifuge – reduces fever.

Fungicidal – kills fungal infections; prevents them from occurring.

Galactagogue – promotes lactation in nursing mothers; increases the secretion of breast milk.

Hemostatic – stops bleeding.

Hepatic – acting on the liver.

Hypertensive – increases blood pressure.

Hypotensive – decreases blood pressure.

Immuno-stimulant – stimulates and strengthens the immune system.

Laxative – facilitate or increase bowel movements.

Mucolytic – helps fluidify mucus in the lungs, making it easier to cough up.

Nervine – strengthens and tones the nerves and the nervous system.

Relaxing – induces calm in the body; has a relaxing effect on body and mind.

Refreshing – to reinvigorate the body; to give new strength or energy to.

Rubefacient – an agent that produces redness of the skin; warms the skin.

Sedative – a substance that reduces mental excitement or irritability, and reduces physical activity.

Soporific –induces drowsiness or sleep.

Stimulant – increases alertness of the mind, and boosts energy.

Stomachic – improves the function of the stomach, increases appetite, and helps with digestion.

Sudorific – increases perspiration.

Tonic – refreshes, revitalizes and invigorates body functions.

Uplifting – lifts the spirits, promotes positive thinking.

Vasoconstrictive – constriction or narrowing of a blood vessel resulting in reduced blood flow to a specific area of the body.

Vasodilatory – the widening of blood vessels resulting in increased blood flow to a specific area of the body.

Vermifuge – expels worms from the intestines.

Vulnerary – a substance which heals wounds.

Warming – produces a feeling of warmth in the body.

5

1,001 Ways to Use
61 Essential Oils

Angelica Root Oil

This oil is great at brightening a dull complexion, and also helps to clear congested skin. Angelica root oil is an excellent detox oil, helping to speed up the removal of wastes and toxins from the body, and for this reason, it is effective at treating arthritis and rheumatism. Colds and flu, along with coughing and bronchitis, can be treated with angelica root oil, while flatulence, indigestion, and nausea are reduced.

Properties: antiseptic, antispasmodic, carminative, cholagogue, depurative, diaphoretic, digestive, diuretic, emmenagogue, expectorant, nervine, stomachic, stimulant, tonic.

Ways to Use Angelica Root Essential Oil

Asthma – angelica root oil helps to calm nerves, which eases breathing. It also clears congestion in the airways. Mix 4 drops with 1 teaspoon of carrier oil, and massage into the chest.

Cellulite – mix 5 drops of the oil with 1 tablespoon of coconut oil, and firmly massage into areas of concern. Angelica root oil contains fantastic diuretic properties, which help to rid the body of toxins and wastes. It also helps to break down fat deposits that build up in the body's tissues.

Detox – angelica root oil is both a detoxifier and diuretic. It helps to purify the blood and remove toxins and excess fluid from the body. Dilute 6 drops in 1 tablespoon of carrier oil, and add to a warm Epsom salt bath.

Digestion – angelica root oil is an excellent tonic for the digestive system as it helps to regulate healthy digestion by stimulating the secretion of digestive juices in the stomach.

Mix 4 drops with 1 teaspoon of carrier oil, and massage into the abdomen in a clockwise direction.

Flatulence – angelica root oil relaxes muscles in the intestines and abdomen, helping to release gases that have built up over time. Mix 4 drops with 1 teaspoon of carrier oil, and massage into the abdomen in a clockwise direction.

Fluid Retention – angelica root oil's ability to increase the frequency and quantity of urination means that it helps to remove excess fluid from the body that may otherwise cause bloating and digestive problems. Mix 4 drops of the oil with 1 teaspoon of carrier oil, and massage into the feet. You can also dilute 6 drops in 1 tablespoon of carrier oil and, add to a warm bath.

Immune System – mix 4 drops with 1 teaspoon of carrier oil, and massage into the feet. Angelica root oil acts as an excellent tonic for the immune system, stimulating and strengthening to prevent illness.

Indecision – angelica root oil is good for those who find it difficult to make decisions and stand up for themselves. It instils strength of character. Diffuse 5 drops in the home, or place 2 drops on a tissue, and inhale regularly.

Irregular Menstruation – angelica root oil promotes regular menstruation and also helps to alleviate the pain of menstrual cramps. Mix 4 drops with 1 teaspoon of carrier oil, and massage into the lower abdomen. For painful cramps, add 3 drops onto a hot compress, and drape across the abdomen for 15 minutes.

Liver Function – mix 4 drops with 1 teaspoon of carrier oil, and massage into the feet. Angelica root oil helps to keep the liver healthy by stimulating the relevant secretions and protecting it from infection. It also helps to free the liver of toxins and wastes.

Loss of Appetite – angelica root oil is said to help with the loss of appetite, which can help in anorexia nervosa cases. Mix 4 drops with 1 teaspoon of carrier oil, and massage into the abdomen in a clockwise direction.

Physical Weakness – whether an individual is weak after being ill, with age, or generally suffers from weakness, angelica root is a beneficial oil to use. It helps to restore strength and stamina, normalizing energy levels in the body.

Rheumatism & Arthritis – the diuretic properties contained within angelica root oil help to ease both rheumatism and arthritis as it is able to eliminate wastes such as uric acids and salt. Mix 4 drops with 1 teaspoon of carrier oil, and massage into painful joints.

Alternatively, place 3-4 drops on a hot compress, and drape over the area of concern for 10 minutes.

Sinusitis – mix 4 drops with 1 teaspoon of carrier oil, and massage into the chest and either side of the nose. Yu can also add 3 drops to a steam inhalation. Angelica root oil clears the respiratory tract of phlegm and mucus and also helps to fight the infection that causes sinusitis.

Stress & Anxiety – angelica root oil has a relaxing effect on the nervous system and helps to calm during times of stress and anxiety. Diffuse 5 drops, or add 15 drops to a 300ml spray mist, and spray around the upper body regularly when needed.

Basil Oil

Basil oil has an uplifting effect on the mind, helping to clear mental fatigue and promote alertness. It is effective at relieving headaches and migraines, clearing sinusitis and bronchitis, and alleviating digestive disorders such as constipation, cramping, vomiting, and flatulence. Basil oil's emmenagogue properties help to regularize menstruation, and in cases where there has been no bleeding, it can stimulate menstruation.

Properties: analgesic, antidepressant, antiseptic, antispasmodic, carminative, digestive, emmenagogue, expectorant, febrifuge, nervine, sudorific, uplifting.

Ways to Use Basil Essential Oil

Acne – basil oil's antibacterial and anti-inflammatory properties make it an effective treatment for acne. Mix 3 drops of basil oil with 1 teaspoon of coconut oil, and massage into the face and neck. Repeat daily.

Amenorrhea (absence of periods) – basil oil is helpful in promoting menstrual flow and should be massaged into the abdomen, lower back, and inner thighs. Mix 4 drops of basil oil with 1 teaspoon of carrier oil. Massage as above, and leave the oils to absorb into the skin.

Anxiety – basil oil's warming and calming properties help to reduce anxiety and any nervous debility. Diffuse 5 drops of the oil, or apply 2 drops on a tissue, and inhale regularly.

Bronchitis – basil oil helps to reduce inflammation of the air passageways and clear infection. Mix 4 drops of the oil with 1 teaspoon of carrier oil, and massage into the front of the neck, chest, and across the top of the shoulders. Repeat daily until symptoms ease.

Depression – basil oil is excellent for uplifting the spirits, therefore instilling feelings of happiness. Diffuse 5 drops, or apply 2 drops to a tissue, and inhale regularly.

Focus & Concentration – diffuse 4 drops of basil oil, or apply 2 drops to a tissue, and inhale regularly. Basil oil helps to focus the mind.

Indigestion – basil oil helps to calm the symptoms of indigestion, particularly where there is too much gas. Mix 4 drops of the oil with 1 teaspoon of carrier oil, and massage into the abdomen using clockwise massage strokes. Repeat daily until the indigestion eases or disappears.

Insect Bites or Stings – basil oil has excellent anti-inflammatory properties, therefore helping to reduce inflammation around insect bites or stings. Mix 3 drops of basil oil with 1 teaspoon of coconut oil, and massage into the bite 2-3 times per day until symptoms ease.

Insomnia – basil oil is an effective oil to use if you suffer from insomnia, particularly if it is due to nervous tension. Place 2 drops on your pillow, or dilute 8 drops in 200ml of water, and place in a spray bottle. Spray onto the pillow before bedtime. Shake well before use.

Mental Fatigue – mix 3 drops of basil oil with 1 teaspoon of carrier oil, and massage into the soles of the feet. Basil oil helps to clear the head, and uplift and stimulate the senses. You can also diffuse 4 drops, and allow the aroma to fill the room.

Migraine – basil oil is an excellent muscle relaxant, therefore it is especially helpful for migraines caused by tension and tight muscles. Diffuse 2 drops of the oil, or mix 2 drops with 1 teaspoon of coconut oil and massage into the back of the neck.

Neuritis – mix 4 drops of basil oil with 1 teaspoon of coconut oil, and massage on either side of the spine from the lower back to the neck area. Basil oil helps to tone the nervous system both physically and emotionally.

Sinusitis – add 3 drops of basil oil to a steam inhalation. Inhale for 2-3 minutes, taking a break if you need to. Alternatively, mix 4 drops of basil oil with 1 teaspoon of carrier oil, and massage into the chest, back of the neck, across the shoulders, and both arms. Basil oil has a positive action on the respiratory tract helping to reduce inflammation and clear mucus.

Stomach Cramps – mix 4 drops of basil oil with 1 teaspoon of carrier oil, and massage into the abdomen and lower back. Basil oil will help to relax and loosen the tight muscles that are causing the cramps.

Tight Muscles – dilute 6 drops of basil oil with 2 tablespoons of carrier oil, and thoroughly massage into tight muscles and surrounding areas. You can also dilute 4 drops of the oil with 1 tablespoon of carrier oil, and add to a warm bath. Soak for 20 minutes. Basil oil helps to loosen and relax muscles due to its strong antispasmodic properties.

Benzoin Oil

This oil has a great calming effect on the nervous and digestive systems, helping to relieve stress and tension, improve digestion, and relieve flatulence. It also has a warming effect on the circulatory system. Benzoin's fantastic anti-inflammatory properties make it an effective healer for sore, wounded skin.

Properties: anti-inflammatory, antiseptic, astringent, carminative, deodorant, expectorant, sedative, vulnerary, warming.

Ways to Use Benzoin Essential Oil

Aging Skin – benzoin's astringent properties help to improve the skin's elasticity, thereby maintaining its shape and firmness. Blend 4 drops with 1 teaspoon of coconut oil, and massage onto the face and neck on a daily basis.

Anxiety – benzoin oil helps to balance the nervous system bringing our emotions under control. As a result, it calms and relaxes the nerves in times of stress or worry. Diffuse 4 drops, or place 2 drops on a tissue, and inhale regularly. Alternatively, blend 5 drops with 1 tablespoon of carrier oil and massage into the chest, neck, across the shoulders, behind the neck and down the arms.

Arthritis – benzoin oil's excellent warming and soothing capabilities means that it is a common ingredient found in arthritis creams and balms. To make your homemade lotion, simply blend 4 drops with 1 teaspoon of carrier oil, and massage into the affected area. If you suffer from arthritis in several places, increase the blend to 7 drops of oil with 2 tablespoons of carrier oil.

Chapped Skin – benzoin oil helps to relieve and heal chapped skin and can prevent any infection from taking place. Mix 3 drops with 1 teaspoon of coconut oil, and massage into the affected area. Repeat twice per day.

Chicken Pox – benzoin oil helps to reduce inflammation and relieve the itching that accompanies chicken pox. Mix 6 drops of the oil with 2 tablespoons of carrier oil, and massage into the body. Repeat once per day for 5 days.

Colds & Flu – add 4 drops to a steam inhalation, and inhale the aroma for 2-3 minutes. Take a break if you need to. Repeat twice per day until symptoms disappear. Benzoin oil possesses impressive expectorant properties, helping to remove any bacteria that might cause a cold or flu. It also clears a congested respiratory tract.

Cracked Heels – mix 4 drops with 1 teaspoon of coconut oil, and massage over and around the heels. Benzoin oil helps to reduce any inflammation on the heels, prevent infection, improve skin elasticity, soothe dry, rough patches of skin around the cracks, and speed up the healing process.

Cystitis – dilute 5 drops in 1 tablespoon of carrier oil, and add to a sitz bath. Sit for 20 minutes. Benzoin oil helps fight infection of the urinary tract.

Deodorant – benzoin oil's sweet vanilla-like fragrance means that it is widely used in the manufacture of deodorants. It is also able to kill the germs responsible for bad body odor. Mix ¼ cup of baking soda with 15 drops of the oil, and apply to the armpits after showering in the morning.

Depression – benzoin oil helps to soothe and stimulate the nervous system, thereby helping to reduce sadness and depression, creating a lift in spirits. Diffuse 4 drops, or place 2 drops on a tissue, and inhale regularly. You can also dilute 6 drops in 1 tablespoon of carrier oil, and add to a warm bath. Repeat every day during times of low moods.

Dermatitis – mix 5 drops of benzoin oil with 1 tablespoon of coconut oil, and massage over the affected area. Benzoin oil has excellent antiseptic properties and is an effective disinfectant. It helps to clear and prevent the spread of dermatitis.

Detox – blend 6 drops with 1 tablespoon of carrier oil, and add to a warm bath (you can also add 1 cup of Epsom salts to further enhance the elimination of toxins). Benzoin oil possesses potent diuretic properties, thereby helping to facilitate the removal of toxins from the blood through urination.

Digestion – benzoin oil acts as a tonic for the digestive system, helping to prevent the build-up of gas in the stomach and intestines, therefore helping to improve digestion. Mix 4 drops with 1 teaspoon of carrier oil, and massage onto the abdomen using circular clockwise movements.

Flatulence – benzoin oil is a powerful carminative and anti-flatulent. It helps to reduce muscle tension in the abdominal area to help expel gas from the stomach and intestines. Mix 4 drops with 1 teaspoon of carrier oil, and massage into the abdomen in a clockwise direction.

PMS – common symptoms of PMS such as irritability, mood swings, depression, and anxiety can be treated using benzoin oil. Simply diffuse 5 drops, and allow the aroma of the oil to circulate around the room and dispel any heavy negative feelings. Also, blend 5 drops with 1 tablespoon of carrier oil, and add to a bath.

Poor Circulation – mix 8 drops with 2 tablespoons of carrier oil, and massage the entire body. Benzoin oil has a warming effect on the body, therefore helping to improve circulation.

Room Freshener – benzoin oil is widely used in the perfume industry due to its sugary vanilla scent. It makes for a beautiful air freshener. Diffuse 5 drops, and allow the scent to fill the room.

Sinusitis – benzoin oil helps to draw out any phlegm or mucus and clear a congested respiratory tract. Add 4 drops to a steam inhalation, and inhale deeply for 2-3 minutes. Repeat as necessary.

Surface Cleaner – benzoin oil contains antibacterial and antiviral components making it an effective oil to use around the home. Place 10 drops of the oil in a spray bottle containing 300ml of water, and spray onto kitchen surfaces to help remove germs and bacteria.

Throat Infections – add 4 drops of benzoin oil to a steam inhalation, and inhale for 2-3 minutes. Take a break if you need to. Benzoin oil contains expectorant properties which help to draw out bacteria that cause the throat infection. It also helps to reduce inflammation of the tissue in the throat area.

Bergamot Oil

A fantastic oil used to promote emotional well being as it helps to release anger and frustration, reduce anxiety and stress, and ease the symptoms of depression. It also contains powerful antiseptic properties, useful for treating skin disorders such as eczema and psoriasis.

Properties: analgesic, antidepressant, antiseptic, antiviral, carminative, cicatrisant, cooling, deodorant, digestive, febrifuge, laxative, relaxing, sedative, stomachic, tonic, vermifuge, vulnerary, uplifting.

Ways to Use Bergamot Essential Oil

Acne – bergamot's antiseptic properties make it a useful treatment for acne as it helps to clear any infection associated with this skin disorder. Mix 3 drops of bergamot oil with 1 teaspoon of coconut oil, and massage into the face and neck. Repeat daily.

Appetite – mix 4 drops of bergamot oil with 1 teaspoon of carrier oil, and massage into the abdomen in clockwise movements. Bergamot oil helps to balance the appetite. May be useful for anorexia nervosa.

Bronchitis – add 3 drops to a steam inhalation, and inhale deeply. You can also mix 4 drops of bergamot with 1 teaspoon of carrier oil, and massage into the chest area. Bergamot oil helps to clear congestion from the lungs.

Confidence – bergamot oil instils feelings of strength and confidence. Apply 2 drops to a tissue, and inhale throughout the day.

Cold Sores – apply 1 neat drop of bergamot oil directly onto a cold sore using a cotton bud, to help heal the infection and speed up the recovery process.

Constipation – bergamot oil helps to stimulate and tone the stomach, helping in cases of constipation. Mix 3 drops with 1 teaspoon of carrier oil, and massage into the lower abdomen in a clockwise direction. Repeat twice per day until symptoms clear.

Cracked Heels – mix 3 drops of bergamot oil with 1 teaspoon of coconut oil, and massage into the heels. Bergamot oil acts as an antiseptic agent, helping to heal the skin.

Cystitis – bergamot oil has an affinity with the urino-genital tract, making it an effective treatment for cystitis and other bladder problems. Dilute 6 drops in 1 tablespoon of carrier oil, and add to a warm sitz bath. Sit for 20 minutes.

Deodorant – mix 1 teaspoon of baking soda with 5 drops of bergamot oil, and apply to the armpits. Bergamot oil creates a natural, citrus smelling deodorant, free from any harsh chemicals.

Depression – bergamot's strong uplifting properties makes it an effective treatment for depression. Apply 2 drops of the oil onto a tissue, and inhale throughout the day. You can also diffuse 5 drops, or mix 4 drops with 1 tablespoon of carrier oil, and massage into the back of the neck, behind the ears, and on the upper chest.

Eczema – bergamot's excellent antiseptic properties means it is a useful treatment for eczema. Mix 2-4 drops with 1 teaspoon of coconut oil, and massage into the affected area. Repeat daily.

Emotional Balance – bergamot oil has excellent uplifting properties, and therefore helps to reduce feelings of anger and frustration. Diffuse 5 drops of the oil, and allow the aroma to fill the room. Alternatively mix 3 drops of bergamot oil with 1 teaspoon of carrier oil, and massage into the chest.

Fever – bergamot oil has a cooling effect on the body, helping to reduce fever and lower body temperature. Add 4 drops to a bowl of cool water, and sponge the body down. You can also diffuse 5 drops of the oil, and allow the aroma to fill the room.

Flatulence – bergamot oil helps to relieve flatulence by regulating the digestive system. Mix 4 drops of the oil with 1 teaspoon of carrier oil, and massage into the lower abdomen in circular clockwise movements.

Muscular Aches & Pains – bergamot oil has powerful analgesic properties and is therefore able to reduce our sensitivity to pain. It is useful in treating any aches and pains, particularly muscular. Dilute 6 drops of bergamot in 1 tablespoon of carrier oil, and add to a warm bath. Soak for 20 minutes. Alternatively, mix 5 drops of the oil with 1 tablespoon of carrier oil, and massage into affected areas.

PMS – bergamot oil helps to create a sense of well being, alleviate low moods, and balance emotions. Diffuse 5 drops of the oil, and allow the room to clear of any negative emotions.

Room Freshener – bergamot oil is often used in the perfume industry because of its delightful scent, and can therefore be used as a natural, air freshener in the home. Diffuse

5 drops of the oil, or apply 3-4 drops on potpourri to keep it smelling fresh, and disperse any unpleasant odors.

Tension & Anxiety – diffuse 5 drops of bergamot oil, or dilute 6 drops in 1 tablespoon of carrier oil, and add to a warm bath. Soak for 20 minutes. Bergamot oil helps to relieve nervous tension and has a relaxing effect on the body and mind.

Thrush – blend 5 drops of bergamot oil with 1 tablespoon of carrier oil, and add to a warm sitz bath. Sit for 20 minutes. Bergamot oil helps to alleviate any discomfort and prevent the spread of infection.

Tonsillitis – bergamot oil is an effective antiseptic for disorders of the respiratory system. Add 3 drops to a steam inhalation, and inhale deeply for 2-3 minutes. Take breaks if you need to. Alternatively mix 3 drops with 1 teaspoon of carrier oil, and massage into the neck and chest.

Birch Oil

With strong pain relieving properties, birch oil is effective at treating rheumatic and arthritic pain, muscular aches and pains, neuralgia, sciatica, and tendonitis. It also helps to reduce inflammation in the above disorders. The appearance of cellulite can be greatly reduced with the use of birch oil, while bloating and water retention are eliminated.

Properties: analgesic, anti-inflammatory, antiseptic, astringent, depurative, disinfectant, diuretic, febrifuge, insecticide, tonic, warming.

Ways to Use Birch Essential Oil

Arthritis & Rheumatism – birch oil acts as a natural pain reliever and can provide relief from joint pain. It also reduces inflammation and stimulates circulation, which can have a positive effect on arthritis and rheumatism.

Cellulite – birch oil helps to reduce the appearance of cellulite over time, as it helps to eliminate toxins and fats from the body due to its diuretic properties. Mix 5 drops with 1 tablespoon of coconut oil, and firmly massage into problem areas.

Detox – mix 4 drops with 1 teaspoon of carrier oil, and massage into the feet. Alternatively, dilute 5 drops in 1 tablespoon of carrier oil, and add to a warm Epsom salt bath. Birch oil has a strong diuretic effect on the body, which results in increased urination and therefore faster elimination of toxins and wastes from the body.

Emotional Support – when you are feeling insecure, unloved or lonely, birch oil can give you strength and help you feel supported. Diffuse 4 drops, or place 2 drops on a tissue, and inhale when needed.

Fever – the febrifuge properties contained within birch oil means it has the ability to cool the body down during fever, giving relief and comfort. Diffuse 4 drops, or add 3 drops to a cold compress, and drape across the forehead or chest.

Headaches – birch oil's analgesic effect is helpful in reducing pain associated with headaches. Mix 2 drops of the oil with 1 teaspoon of coconut oil, and massage into the temples and back of the neck.

Muscular Aches & Pains – aching muscles can be relieved with the use of birch oil due to its anti-inflammatory, pain relieving, and warming properties. Mix 5 drops with 1 tablespoon of carrier oil, and massage into the areas of concern. Alternatively, dilute 5 drops in 1 tablespoon of carrier oil, and add to a warm bath.

Poor Circulation – birch oil helps to stimulate blood circulation, helping to improve the delivery of nutrients around the body, reduce the appearance of varicose veins, and alleviate edema. Mix 4 drops with 1 teaspoon of carrier oil, and massage into the soles of the feet.

Tendonitis – mix 2-3 drops with 1 teaspoon of carrier oil, and massage into the area of concern. Birch oil helps to reduce inflammation around tendons and also eases pain.

Warming – birch oil is a very warming and comforting oil and can be particularly beneficial when used in the winter months to ease aches and pains, ward off colds and flu, and stimulate circulation, Diffuse 4 drops in your home.

Black Pepper Oil

A great companion for the digestive system as it helps to improve sluggish digestion. It is a great warming oil thus relieving muscular aches and pains. It also helps to combat poor circulation.

Properties: analgesic, antiseptic, antispasmodic, carminative, diaphoretic, diuretic, febrifuge, laxative, rubefacient, stomachic, tonic.

Ways to Use Black Pepper Essential Oil

Arthritis – black pepper oil's warming and pain relieving properties help to successfully treat rheumatic and arthritic pain. Mix 3 drops with 1 teaspoon of carrier oil, and massage into areas of concern.

Colds & Flu – mix 3 drops with 1 teaspoon of carrier oil, and massage into the chest to help warm the body and fight off the infection.

Constipation – black pepper oil helps to relieve constipation by stimulating the large intestines and encouraging peristalsis. Mix 3 drops with 1 teaspoon of carrier oil, and massage into the abdomen in a clockwise direction.

Detox – mix 3 drops with 1 teaspoon of carrier oil, and massage into the feet. Black pepper oil promotes sweating and increases the duration and frequency of urination which helps to get rid of toxins and wastes from the body.

Digestion – black pepper oil is a valuable oil for treating sluggish digestion as it stimulates the secretion of digestive juices and bile that allow efficient digestion to take place. Mix 3 drops with 1 teaspoon of carrier oil, and massage over the abdomen in a clockwise direction.

Memory Loss – diffusing 3 drops of black pepper oil helps to enhance concentration and improve memory loss.

Nausea – place 2 drops of black pepper oil on a tissue, and inhale each time you feel pangs of nausea.

Pre Exercise – black pepper oil is believed to improve exercise performance or training due to its ability to prevent pain and stiffness in muscles. Mix 4 drops with 1 tablespoon of carrier oil, and massage into large muscle groups before working out.

Poor Circulation – black pepper oil's warming action on the body helps to stimulate circulation. Mix 3 drops with 1 teaspoon of carrier oil, and massage into the feet.

Stiff, Tight Muscles – black pepper oil has a wonderful warming effect on stiff muscles, helping to loosen muscles and ease aches and pains. Mix 4 drops with 1 tablespoon of carrier oil, and massage into affected muscles. You can also dilute 4 drops in 1 tablespoon of carrier oil, and add to a warm bath.

Cajeput Oil

Cajeput oil has an affinity with the respiratory system, effectively clearing air passageways by expelling mucus from the lungs and clearing congestion from the nasal passageways. It is a useful oil to use during times of fever as it helps to cool the body down and fight infection. As a digestive aid, cajeput oil eases vomiting, nausea, indigestion, and dysentery.

Properties: analgesic, antiseptic, antispasmodic, expectorant, febrifuge, stimulant, sudorific, vermifuge.

Ways to Use Cajeput Essential Oil

Arthritis & Rheumatism – mix 3 drops with 1 teaspoon of carrier oil, and massage into the areas of concern. Cajeput oil reduces the sensation of pain and also helps reduce any swelling around joints.

Cuts & Wounds – mix 3 drops with 1 teaspoon of carrier oil, and massage over the affected area twice per day. Cajeput oil helps to clean the wound and prevent any infection from taking place.

Fatigue – cajeput oil acts as a stimulant for the nervous system, helping to energize and invigorate a fatigued mind and body. Add 10 drops to a spray mist, and spray over the upper body regularly. You can also diffuse 3 drops in your home.

Fever – cajeput oil helps to cool down body temperature during fever and contains antimicrobial properties which help to fight the infection that caused the fever. Mix 3 drops with 1 teaspoon of carrier oil, and massage into the chest area, or add 2 drops to a steam inhalation.

Influenza – cajeput oil helps to clear the influenza virus and ease congestion and mucus build up. Add 2 drops to a steam inhalation, or mix 3 drops with 1 teaspoon of carrier oil, and massage into the chest area.

Insect Repellent – diffusing 3 drops of cajeput oil makes for an excellent insect repellent, helping to keep mosquitoes and bugs away.

Sciatica – cajeput oil has excellent pain relieving properties that make it a beneficial oil to treat sciatica. Mix 4 drops with 1 tablespoon of carrier oil, and massage the entire leg and buttock region.

Sinusitis – cajeput oil helps to clear congested nasal passageways and ease breathing. Add 3 drops to a steam inhalation, or mix 3 drops with 1 teaspoon of carrier oil, and massage into the chest area.

Sore Throat – gargle a small amount of water with 2 drops of cajeput oil. Do not swallow. Cajeput oil helps to reduce an inflamed throat and ease any pain or discomfort.

Toothache – cajeput oil helps to dull the pain of a toothache and reduce an inflamed gum. Mix 2 drops with ½ teaspoon of carrier oil, and massage into the gum where the pain can be felt. Repeat twice per day.

Carrot Seed Oil

Carrot seed oil is an excellent tonic for the skin, helping to improve tone and elasticity, reduce fine lines and wrinkles, treat eczema and psoriasis, and balance sebum production in oily skin. Water retention and cellulite can be successfully treated using carrot seed oil, while its tonic action on the liver and gall bladder is used to detoxify the body and alleviate jaundice.

Properties: antiseptic, carminative, cytophylactic, depurative, diuretic, emmenagogue, hepatic, stimulant, tonic, vermifuge.

Ways to Use Carrot Seed Essential Oil

Anti-Aging – carrot seed oil contains powerful antioxidant properties, which help to fight free radicals in the skin. These free radicals damage healthy tissue and destroy skin cells that will eventually lead to premature aging. Mix 5 drops with 1 teaspoon of coconut oil, and massage into the face and neck. Repeat twice per day.

Detox – carrot seed oil has excellent detoxifying capabilities and works well at clearing toxins from the blood, body tissues, muscles, joints, and liver. Mix 4 drops with 1 teaspoon of carrier oil, and massage into the feet. You can also dilute 6 drops in 1 tablespoon of carrier oil, and add to a warm Epsom salt bath. Repeat daily for 1 week.

Eczema – carrot seed oil helps to ease itchy skin and reduce inflammation. Mix 3 drops with 1 teaspoon of coconut oil, and massage over the affected area.

Flatulence – mix 4 drops with 1 teaspoon of carrier oil, and massage into the abdomen in a clockwise direction. Carrot seed oil helps to inhibit the formation of gas in the intestines.

Fluid Retention – carrot seed oil helps to prevent or reduce fluid retention due to its diuretic properties. Mix 8 drops with 2 tablespoons of carrier oil, and massage into the body. For specific areas of fluid retention, mix 4 drops with 1 teaspoon of carrier oil, and massage into the affected areas using upward strokes towards the heart.

Gout – carrot seed oil helps to rid the body of uric acid which can cause gout. Mix 4 drops with 1 teaspoon of carrier oil, and massage into the area of concern. Repeat twice per day.

Immune System – mix 4 drops with 1 teaspoon of carrier oil, and massage into the soles of the feet. Carrot seed oil contains antiseptic, antiviral, and antioxidant qualities, which enhance the immune system, thereby protecting it from illness.

Irregular Menstruation – carrot seed oil balances the hormones of the female reproductive system, therefore regulating the menstrual cycle. Mix 4 drops with 1 teaspoon of carrier oil, and massage into the abdomen in a clockwise direction.

Mental Alertness – carrot seed oil stimulates the nervous system, which in turn stimulates the activity of the brain, making you more alert and focused. Diffuse 5 drops, or place 3 drops on a tissue, and inhale throughout the day.

Well Being – diffusing 5 drops of carrot seed oil in the home helps to release negative energy and enhance feelings of well being.

Cedarwood Oil

An effective oil in balancing both dry and oily skin conditions, cedarwood oil also helps to cleanse the skin of any impurities, and is also a popular choice for treating dandruff. Its role as a diuretic makes it a valuable oil to treat cellulite, fluid retention, and the accumulation of toxins in the blood.

Properties: antiseborrheic, antiseptic, antispasmodic, astringent, diuretic, emmenagogue, expectorant, fungicide, insecticide, sedative, tonic.

Ways to Use Cedarwood Essential Oil

Acne – cedarwood oil helps to regulate sebum production and has excellent antibacterial and antiseptic properties, making it an ideal oil to use on acne. Mix 4 drops of the oil with 1 teaspoon of coconut oil, and massage into the face and neck.

Anxiety – apply 3 drops of the oil onto a tissue, and inhale throughout the day. Cedarwood oil helps to reduce anxiety and calm the mind.

Bladder Infection – blend 4 drops of cedarwood oil with 1 tablespoon of carrier oil, and massage into the abdomen and lower back. Cedarwood oil is an excellent tonic for the urinary system and can help clear bladder infections.

Cellulite – cedarwood oil is a fantastic treatment for cellulite as it helps to decongest sluggish tissues, drawing out any excess fat in between the tissues. Mix 6 drops of the oil with 1 tablespoon of coconut oil, and massage into affected areas. Repeat daily for excellent results.

Coughing – adding 3 drops of cedarwood oil to a steam inhalation helps to clear air passageways by breaking up and expelling mucus in the respiratory tract.

Cystitis – cedarwood oil helps to relieve any pain and inflammation associated with cystitis. Dilute 4-6 drops in 1 tablespoon of carrier oil, and add to a warm bath. Soak for 20 minutes. Alternatively, mix 4 drops of the oil with 1 teaspoon of carrier oil, and massage into the lower abdomen in a clockwise direction.

Dandruff – mix 6 drops of cedarwood oil to 1 tablespoon of olive oil, and massage into the scalp. Leave for 30 minutes and rinse. Alternatively, add 5 drops to your shampoo when washing your hair.

Fluid Retention – mix 7 drops of cedarwood oil with 2 tablespoons of coconut oil, and massage into the body. Alternatively, mix 3 drops with 1 teaspoon of coconut oil, and massage into the soles of the feet. Cedarwood oil is a mild diuretic, and therefore helps to combat and reduce fluid retention.

Hair Loss – mix 3 drops of cedarwood oil with 1 teaspoon of carrier oil, and rub into a bald spot to promote new hair growth twice daily. Regular use is advised to produce successful results.

Insomnia – mix 5 drops of the oil with 1 teaspoon of carrier oil, and massage into the feet before bedtime to help overcome broken sleep or insomnia. Alternatively, place 2 drops onto your pillow.

Insect Repellent – diffuse 5 drops of cedarwood oil, and place in a safe place to repel any pesky insects. Alternatively, add 12 drops of the oil to a 200ml spray bottle filled with filtered water, and spray around the upper and lower body regularly.

Mental Clarity – diffuse 4 drops of cedarwood oil, and allow the aroma to fill the room. This oil promotes focus and calm, and helps to improve attention and concentration. Alternatively, mix 2 drops with 1 teaspoon of carrier oil, and massage the formula into the back of the neck.

Muscular Spasms – cedarwood oil has a calming, balancing effect on muscles, and should be massaged into the affected area daily to reduce spasms. Mix 5 drops of the oil with 1 tablespoon of carrier oil, and massage into the affected muscle. Cedarwood oil's warming properties will also help relieve muscular aches and pains.

Pore Size – blend 4 drops of cedarwood oil with 1 teaspoon of coconut oil, and massage into the face, focusing on the upper cheeks, nose, forehead, and chin. Cedarwood oil's astringent properties help to tighten and tone pores.

Stress – cedarwood oil's warm and gentle action on the body and mind makes it a great treatment for stress and tension. Diffuse 4 drops of the oil, or place 2 drops on a tissue, and inhale regularly, particularly in times of stressful situations.

Chamomile (Roman) Oil

Roman chamomile is an excellent calming and relaxing oil. It is great for soothing inflammation and relieving pain from aches and pains, particularly muscular. It is a beneficial oil to use for dry skin conditions such as eczema, dermatitis, and psoriasis. Roman Chamomile acts as a tonic for the digestive system, helping to relieve flatulence, gastritis, and diarrhea. It reduces irritability and lessens anxiety.

Properties: analgesic, anti-inflammatory, antiseptic, antispasmodic, bactericidal, carminative, cholagogue, digestive, emmenagogue, febrifuge, hepatic, sedative, stomachic, sudorific, vermifuge, vulnerary, tonic.

Ways to Use Chamomile (Roman) Essential Oil

Acne – chamomile (Roman) helps to clear acne by removing toxins and bacteria from sebaceous glands. It also reduces any inflammation that can accompany this skin disorder. Mix 4 drops with 1 teaspoon of coconut oil, and massage into the face and neck. Leave on the skin to absorb. Repeat daily.

Allergies – chamomile oil (Roman) offers excellent relief to those suffering from allergies as it helps to soothe irritated and inflamed nasal passageways. Place 3 drops on a tissue, and inhale regularly throughout the day.

Anger – the beautiful fresh scent of Roman chamomile infuses the air with feelings of tranquillity, calm, and peace, and therefore helps to alleviate anger and frustration. Diffuse 6 drops of the oil, or place 10 drops in a spray bottle filled with 300ml of water, and spray over the body regularly. Shake well before use.

Children – chamomile oil (Roman) is gentle enough to use on babies and children. You should always dilute the oil, and only use a small number of drops. For a baby, mix 1-2 drops (2-3 drops for a child) with 1 teaspoon (1 tablespoon for a child) of coconut oil, and massage onto the legs, arms, and trunk of the body. It can be used to induce calmness, help relieve nappy rash, soothe toothaches or earaches, relieve colic, fight fevers, and alleviate aches and pains.

Constipation – mix 4 drops with 1 teaspoon of carrier oil, and massage into the abdomen and lower back. Roman chamomile oil helps to facilitate bowel movements and reduce any inflammation that may be preventing a bowel movement from taking place.

Depression – chamomile oil (Roman) helps to lift our spirits, encouraging feelings of joy and happiness, and eliminating feelings of despair, sadness, and loneliness. Diffuse 6 drops of the oil, or simply place 3 drops on a tissue, and inhale regularly. You can also dilute 7 drops in 1 tablespoon of carrier oil, and add to a warm bath.

Detox – as a diuretic, Roman chamomile helps to stimulate increased urination, thereby flushing the body of toxins at a faster rate. Blend 6 drops with 1 tablespoon of carrier oil, and add to a warm bath (add 1 cup of Epsom salts to further enhance the detoxification process).

Diarrhea – mix 5 drops with 1 teaspoon of carrier oil, and massage into the abdomen. Roman chamomile acts as a tonic for the digestive system and helps to relieve diarrhea.

Flatulence – mix 5 drops with 1 tablespoon of carrier oil, and massage into the abdomen in circular, clockwise movements. Roman chamomile provides relief from gas in the digestive tract and also prevents the build up of gas, which can cause a sluggish digestion.

Hay Fever – chamomile oil (Roman) helps to calm and soothe the symptoms of hay fever such as itchy eyes, runny nose, and puffy skin. Mix 3 drops with 1 teaspoon of coconut oil, and massage into the face. You can also place 3 drops on a tissue, and inhale regularly, or diffuse 5 drops in a room. Repeat regularly.

Insomnia – place 2 drops on your pillow, or diffuse 4 drops before bedtime. Roman chamomile's calming and sedative properties will ensure you get a good night's sleep.

Menstrual Cramps – chamomile (Roman) oil's valuable antispasmodic properties makes this oil an effective treatment for menstrual cramps as it helps to reduce muscle spasms that cause the cramps. Mix 5 drops with 1 teaspoon of carrier oil, and massage into the abdomen and lower back.

Nausea – chamomile (Roman) helps to relax the smooth muscles which line the stomach and intestines, thereby relieving nausea. Mix 5 drops with 1 teaspoon of carrier oil, and massage into the abdomen. Repeat twice per day as necessary.

PMS – irritability, depression, nervous tension, and anger experienced during PMS can be greatly reduced when you diffuse 6 drops of the oil as soon as you feel the onset of any of the symptoms.

Clary Sage Oil

Clary sage is valuable in balancing hormones, helping to relieve symptoms of PMS, easing menstrual cramps, and alleviating menopausal symptoms. It is also deeply relaxing and euphoric, promoting feelings of well being. Its antispasmodic properties make it effective in easing the symptoms of asthma.

Properties: aphrodisiac, antidepressant, anti-inflammatory, antispasmodic, deodorant, emmenagogue, hypotensive, nervine, relaxing, sedative, tonic, uplifting, warming.

Ways to Use Clary Sage Essential Oil

Creativity – clary sage helps to promote creativity by focusing the mind, putting things into perspective, and creating inspirational thoughts. Diffuse 5 drops in your home.

Dandruff – mix 7 drops with 1 tablespoon of olive or coconut oil, and massage into the scalp. Leave for 20 minutes and then wash hair as normal. Clary sage has an invigorating effect on the scalp.

Depression – clary sage has excellent antidepressant capabilities, being able to induce feelings of optimism, joy, hope, and happiness. It uplifts spirits and helps to create a positive outlook on life. Diffuse 4 drops in your home to clear the air of negative energy, or mix 4 drops with 1 teaspoon of carrier oil, and massage over the heart area.

Digestion – clary sage oil acts as a tonic for the stomach and digestive system. It helps to promote the efficient absorption of nutrients, normalize the secretion of digestive juices, and alleviate stomach problems. Mix 4 drops with 1 teaspoon of carrier oil, and massage into the abdomen in a clockwise direction.

High Blood Pressure – dilute 4 drops of clary sage oil with 1 tablespoon of carrier oil, and add to a warm bath. You can also mix 3 drops with 1 teaspoon of carrier oil, and massage over the heart area. Clary sage relaxes and widens blood vessels, thereby promoting and maintaining regular blood circulation.

Insomnia – clary sage is both sedative and relaxing in nature, having a calming effect on the mind so as to induce a good night's sleep. Place 2 drops on your pillow before bedtime, or diffuse 4 drops in your bedroom about 15 minutes before retiring for bed.

Menopause – clary sage oil regulates female hormones, helps boost mental strength, alleviates low moods, fights depression, and reduces bloating. Dilute 5 drops in 1 tablespoon of carrier oil, and add to a warm bath. You can also diffuse 4 drops, or mix 4 drops with 1 teaspoon of carrier oil, and massage into the feet.

Menstrual Cramps – clary sage oil relieves painful menstruation as it helps to ease spasms in the uterus. Mix 4 drops with 1 teaspoon of carrier oil, and massage into the abdomen in a clockwise direction.

Migraines – relief from migraine headaches can be obtained by using clary sage oil, as it promotes blood circulation, and also has a sedative, gentle effect on the brain. Mix 2 drops with ½ teaspoon of coconut oil, and massage into the temples.

Muscle Cramps – clary sage is a powerful muscle relaxant and its antispasmodic qualities help to ease the painful tightening of muscles, which can result in cramps. Mix 4 drops with 1 teaspoon of carrier oil, and massage into the area of concern. Alternatively, dilute 5 drops with 1 tablespoon of carrier oil, and add to a warm bath.

Oily Hair – clary sage oil helps to balance excess sebum production in the scalp, reducing the possibility of oily hair. Add 4 drops to 1 ounce of conditioner, and leave for 10 minutes. Rinse and style as normal.

Oily Skin – clary sage oil helps to regenerate the skin, increase skin tone by improving a sluggish circulation, and balance excess sebum production in skin cells, which helps to alleviate oily skin and prevent breakouts. Mix 3 drops with 1 teaspoon of coconut oil, and massage into the face and neck. Repeat daily.

PMS – dilute 5 drops in 1 tablespoon of carrier oil, and add to a warm bath. You can also diffuse 4 drops of oil, or add 10 drops to a 300ml spray bottle filled with filtered water, and spray around the upper body when you feel the need. Shake well before use. Clary sage oil helps to balance the hormones of the female reproductive system. It also treats the emotional problems that accompany PMS by instilling feelings of joy and euphoria.

Poor Circulation – clary sage oil helps to counteract a sluggish circulation and improve the transport of blood around the body. Dilute 5 drops of the oil in 1 tablespoon of carrier oil, and add to a warm bath. Follow up with a cool shower for 20 seconds to further boost circulation.

Stress & Anxiety – clary sage oil provides great relief and comfort in times of stress or tension as it is a powerful muscular relaxant and has a profound soothing effect on the mind. Place 3 drops on a tissue, and inhale regularly, or diffuse 4 drops in your home to clear the air. You can also mix 4 drops with 1 teaspoon of carrier oil, and massage into the upper chest, back of the neck, and across the shoulders.

Varicose Veins – regular massage, using clary sage, oil helps to improve the appearance of varicose veins by promoting blood circulation around the body. Mix 4 drops of the oil with 1 tablespoon of carrier oil, and massage the entire limb in the direction of the heart. Never massage directly over varicose veins, gently massage on either side.

Coriander Oil

Coriander oil has a stimulating effect on digestion, helping to improve the passage of foods and nutrients through the digestive tract. It promotes the appetite thus helping individuals suffering from anorexia nervosa. Its warming action makes it ideal for treating joint pain and neuralgia. Coriander oil has a revitalizing effect on the mind, helping to lift mental fatigue and promote focus and concentration.

Properties: analgesic, antispasmodic, aphrodisiac, bactericidal, carminative, depurative, digestive, fungicidal, stimulant, stomachic.

Ways to Use Coriander Essential Oil

Anorexia Nervosa – coriander oil stimulates the appetite and is therefore helpful in treating anorexia nervosa. Mix 4 drops with 1 teaspoon of carrier oil, and massage into the abdomen in a clockwise direction.

Aphrodisiac – coriander oil helps to increase sexual desire and libido, having a positive effect on a couple's sex life. Diffuse 4 drops in your home, or mix 4 drops with 1 teaspoon of carrier oil, and massage into the feet.

Athlete's Foot – mix 3 drops with 1 teaspoon of coconut oil, and massage into the infection, making sure to massage in between the toes. Coriander oil has excellent fungicidal properties which help to kill the fungus that causes athlete's foot.

Cellulite – coriander oil has a stimulating effect on circulation and also helps to eliminate fluid retention, therefore having a positive effect on reducing the appearance of cellulite. Mix 5 drops with 1 tablespoon of coconut oil, and firmly massage into areas of concern. Repeat 3-4 times per week.

Depression – coriander oil promotes feelings of well being, happiness, and joy, and also helps to provide a sense of security and sense of worth. Diffuse 4 drops, or mix 4 drops with 1 teaspoon of carrier oil, and massage over the heart area.

Detox – dilute 6 drops of coriander oil with 1 tablespoon of carrier oil, and add to a warm Epsom salt bath. Coriander oil helps to purify the blood, cleansing it of toxins and wastes.

Digestion – coriander oil helps to maintain a healthy digestion by stimulating the secretion of digestive juices and relieving flatulence. Mix 4 drops with 1 teaspoon of carrier oil, and massage into the abdomen in a clockwise direction.

Headaches – the analgesic properties contained within coriander oil make it an effective treatment for headaches. Mix 2 drops with 1 teaspoon of carrier oil, and massage into the temples, forehead, and back of the neck.

Impotency – coriander oil reputedly assists in overcoming male or female impotency, while easing any worries or fears that may accompany the problem. Mix 4 drops with 1 teaspoon of carrier oil, and massage into the feet. You can also diffuse 4 drops in the bedroom, or place 1 drop on each pillow before bedtime.

Joint Pain – coriander oil contains pain relieving and warming properties, which together, help to ease stiff and painful joints. Mix 4 drops with 1 teaspoon of carrier oil, and massage into affected areas.

Low Energy – coriander oil has an invigorating effect on the nervous system and helps to stimulate energy levels. Place 2 drops on a tissue, and inhale regularly. Alternatively, add 10 drops to a 300ml spray bottle filled with filtered water, and spray over the head and upper body when needed. Shake well before use.

Mental Fatigue – diffusing 4 drops of coriander oil will help to invigorate the mind and ease mental fatigue.

Muscular Aches & Pains – muscular aches and pains can be reduced by the antispasmodic and analgesic properties of coriander oil. Dilute 6 drops in 1 tablespoon of carrier oil, and add to a warm bath. You can also mix 5 drops with 1 tablespoon of carrier oil, and massage into sore muscles.

PMS – coriander oil helps to calm irritability and stress often felt during PMS and also promotes estrogen production, creating hormonal balance. Mix 4 drops with 1 teaspoon of carrier oil, and massage into the feet. You can also diffuse 4 drops of clear negative energy.

Stomach Health – mix 4 drops with 1 teaspoon of carrier oil, and massage into the upper abdomen in a clockwise direction. Coriander oil acts as an overall tonic for the stomach, helping to reduce cramps and tone the stomach.

Cypress Oil

Cypress oil's astringent and detoxification properties make this oil an excellent choice for use on oily skin as it helps to tighten the pores, control the production of oil in the skin, combat excessive perspiration, and control water loss. It is also an excellent tonic for cellulite and fluid retention.

Properties: antiseptic, antispasmodic, astringent, deodorant, diuretic, hemostatic, hepatic, sudorific, tonic, uplifting, vasoconstrictive.

Ways to Use Cypress Essential Oil

Asthma – cypress oil helps to reduce muscle spasms and sedate nerve endings of the respiratory system, thereby lessening the chances of an asthma attack. Diffuse 4 drops of the oil.

Bleeding Gums – cypress oil helps to slow the flow of excessive bleeding. Place 2 drops in a small glass of water, and use as a mouth rinse. Do not swallow.

Cellulite – mix 6 drops of cypress oil with 1 tablespoon of carrier oil, and massage into the affected area using gentle but firm pressure. Repeat daily. Cypress oil has powerful astringent and diuretic properties.

Coughs – cypress oil helps to relax the nerve endings of the respiratory system and expel mucus. Place 4 drops in a diffuser, and allow the clearing aroma to fill the room.

Cystitis – Dilute 4 drops in 1 tablespoon of carrier oil, and add to a warm sitz bath. Cypress oil will help to speed up the recovery of cystitis as it has powerful diuretic properties.

Dandruff – cypress oil is a useful treatment for dandruff as it helps to regulate the production of oil in the skin. Mix 6 drops with 1 tablespoon of carrier oil, and massage into the scalp. Leave to absorb into the scalp for 1 hour, and rinse thoroughly. Repeat 2-3 times per week.

Diarrhea – mix 4 drops with 1 tablespoon of carrier oil, and massage into the abdomen using clockwise, circular movements. Cypress oil helps to decrease the excessive flow of fluids.

Edema – perhaps best known for its positive effects on any form of fluid retention, cypress oil is a particularly useful oil to use for treating edema. Mix 6 drops with 1 tablespoon of carrier oil, and massage over the affected area. Always massage using gentle pressure in an upwards motion towards the heart.

Emotional Upset – cypress oil has a soothing effect on the nervous system, helping to restore calm and stop crying spells. Diffuse 5 drops of the oil, or place 2 drops on a tissue and inhale regularly.

Excessive Perspiration – dilute 5 drops in 1 tablespoon of carrier oil, and add to a warm bath. Soak for 15 to 20 minutes. Alternatively mix 8 drops with 2 tablespoons of carrier oil, and massage over the entire body. Use coconut oil if massaging onto the face. Regular treatment with cypress oil will ease excessive perspiration considerably.

Fluid Retention – cypress oil has excellent diuretic properties and is an ideal oil to use when suffering from fluid retention. Mix 6 drops with 1 tablespoon of carrier oil, and massage over the affected area always in the direction of the heart. Repeat twice per day until symptoms ease.

Heavy Menstruation – cypress oil helps to contract blood vessels due to its powerful astringent properties and, as a result, helps to reduce abnormally heavy menstruation. Mix 4 drops with 1 tablespoon of carrier oil, and massage into the abdomen and lower back.

Hemorrhoids – cypress oil provides relief from hemorrhoids by constricting blood vessels, improving circulation, releasing toxins from the body, and strengthening connective tissue. Dilute 5 drops in 1 tablespoon of carrier oil, and add to a warm sitz bath. Soak for 20 minutes. Repeat 3-4 times per week.

Hot Flashes – cypress oil contains soothing and cooling properties and also helps to balance the female reproductive system, making it a beneficial oil to treat the symptoms of menopause. Blend 5 drops of the oil in 1 tablespoon of carrier oil, and add to a warm bath. Soak for 20 minutes. You can also diffuse 5 drops to cool the body down.

Menstrual Cramps – mix 5 drops of cypress oil with 1 tablespoon of carrier oil, and massage into the abdomen and lower back. Cypress oil helps to reduce muscular spasms which cause menstrual cramps.

Nose Bleeding – mix 4 drops of cypress oil with 1 teaspoon of carrier oil, and massage into the back of the neck, behind the ears and, into the sides of the nose. Cypress oil helps to reduce excessive bleeding and can be a very beneficial oil to use when suffering from regular nose bleeds.

Oily Skin – due to its astringent properties, cypress oil is an excellent choice to use on oily skin. Dilute 4 drops with 1 teaspoon of coconut oil, and massage into the face. Leave the oils to absorb into the skin. Repeat daily.

PMS – diffusing 5 drops of cypress oil helps to ease some of the symptoms of PMS as it helps to balance the female reproductive system and restore emotional upset.

Poor Circulation – dilute 5 drops in 1 tablespoon of carrier oil, and add to a warm bath. Soak for 20 minutes. You can also blend 8 drops with 2 tablespoons of carrier oil, and massage the body, always towards the direction of the heart. Cypress oil helps to improve sluggish circulation.

Post Exercise – cypress oil helps to ease tension in the muscles and reduce pain, making it a suitable oil to use after a workout. Mix 6 drops of the oil with 1 tablespoon of carrier oil, and massage into large muscle groups in the thighs, back, abdominals, and upper arms.

Stress & Tension – diffuse 5 drops, and allow the sedative nature of cypress oil to fill the room. It helps to induce a calm, relaxed effect on the body and mind. You can also dilute 5 drops in 1 tablespoon of carrier oil, and add to a warm bath.

Sweaty Feet – cypress oil is extremely beneficial at regulating foot odors as it is able to cool the feet and significantly reduce excessive perspiration. Mix 4 drops of the oil with 1 teaspoon of light, non greasy carrier oil, and massage into the feet and ankles, making sure to massage in between the toes.

Swollen Feet – cypress oil aims to improve poor circulation, helping to ease tired, swollen feet. Dilute 4 drops in 1 teaspoon of carrier oil, and add to a warm foot bath. Soak for 20 minutes and repeat regularly.

Varicose Veins – mix 4 drops of cypress oil with 1 teaspoon of carrier oil, and massage the affected limb, making sure to massage on either side of the varicose vein, never directly over it. Always massage in the direction of the heart. Cypress oil is a fantastic choice oil for treating varicose veins as it helps to stimulate a sluggish circulation, constrict blood vessels and has a detoxifying effect on the entire body.

Weak Bladder – when used on a regular basis, cypress oil helps to reduce the excessive flow of urine. Mix 4 drops with 1 tablespoon of carrier oil, and massage into the abdomen and lower back.

Elemi Oil

With an excellent rejuvenating effect on the skin, elemi oil helps to reduce wrinkles and scar tissue, it reduces the appearance of stretch marks, and helps to heal chapped skin. It is effective at clearing respiratory complaints such as coughing, bronchitis, and colds and flu. Elemi oil has a wonderful balancing effect on the emotions and is useful for anyone suffering from stress or tension.

Properties: analgesic, antiseptic, cicatrisant, expectorant, stimulant, stomachic, tonic.

Ways to Use Elemi Essential Oil

Aging Skin – elemi oil helps to reduce fine lines and wrinkles, and also helps to improve skin tone. Mix 4 drops with 1 teaspoon of coconut oil, and massage into the face and neck.

Athlete's Foot – mix 4 drops with 1 teaspoon of coconut oil, and massage into the problem area, making sure to massage in between the toes. Alternatively, add 4 drops to a foot bath, and soak for 20 minutes.

Bronchitis – elemi oil possesses excellent expectorant properties, helping to ease congestion and clear mucus. Mix 4 drops with 1 teaspoon of carrier oil, and massage into the chest area, or add 3 drops to a steam inhalation.

Chapped, Cracked Skin – mix 4 drops with 1 teaspoon of coconut oil, and massage into the area twice per day. Elemi oil encourages new skin cell formation and normalizes dry skin.

Coughing – elemi oil is effective at loosening and removing a build up of mucus in the respiratory tract. Add 3 drops to a steam inhalation, or mix 4 drops with 1 teaspoon of carrier oil, and massage into the chest.

Cuts & Wounds – mix 3 drops with 1 teaspoon of coconut oil, and massage over the area of concern twice per day. Elemi oil has excellent antiseptic properties and is capable of healing wounds and preventing them from becoming infected.

Cystitis – elemi oil acts as a tonic for the urinary tract, protecting it against infection and helping to clear infection when present. Dilute 5 drops in 1 tablespoon of carrier oil, and add to a warm bath.

Immunity – elemi oil acts as a tonic for the immune system, revitalizing and strengthening the body's systems. Dilute 6 drops in 1 tablespoon of carrier oil, and add to a warm bath. Alternatively, mix 4 drops with 1 teaspoon of carrier oil, and massage into the feet.

Muscular & Joint Pain – elemi oil is a beneficial treatment for muscular aches and pains, or joint pains due to its potent pain relieving properties. Mix 5 drops with 1 tablespoon of carrier oil, and massage into the areas of concern. Alternatively, you can dilute 6 drops in 1 tablespoon of carrier oil, and add to a warm bath.

Rashes – mix 3 drops (5-6 for larger areas) with 1 teaspoon (1-2 tablespoons for larger areas), and massage over the area of concern. Elemi oil helps to soothe any inflammation and clear the rash, preventing it from becoming infected.

Scar Tissue – elemi oil's ability to encourage the growth of new skin cells makes it an effective treatment for scar tissue. Mix 3 drops with 1 teaspoon of coconut oil, and gently massage over the area of concern twice per day.

Stress – elemi oil has a calming effect on the body and mind, encouraging harmony and peacefulness. Diffuse 4 drops, or place 2 drops on a tissue, and inhale regularly when needed.

Mature Skin – elemi oil has a rejuvenating effect on mature skin due to its cell regenerating properties. Mix 4 drops with 1 teaspoon of coconut oil, and massage into the face and neck.

Nervous Exhaustion – elemi oil helps to calm the nerves and revitalize a tired mind. Diffuse 4 drops, or dilute 5 drops in 1 tablespoon of carrier oil, and add to a warm bath.

Sinusitis – elemi oil helps to clear congestion in the sinuses, making breathing easier. Add 3 drops to a steam inhalation, or mix 4 drops with 1 teaspoon of carrier oil, and massage into the sides of the nose and chest area.

Eucalyptus Globulus Oil

This oil is effective for treating a number of respiratory disorders such as throat infections, sinusitis, asthma, cough, and symptoms of colds & flu. Eucalyptus oil stimulates and strengthens the immune system by protecting against infection. It also helps to ease muscular aches and pains.

Properties: analgesic, antibacterial, anti-inflammatory, antirheumatic, antiseptic, antispasmodic, antiviral, astringent, cicatrisant, decongestant, deodorant, diuretic, expectorant, febrifuge, insecticide, rubefacient, vermifuge, vulnerary.

Ways to Use Eucalyptus Globulus Essential Oil

Arthritis – eucalyptus oil helps to soothe pain experienced with arthritis, while its anti-inflammatory qualities help to reduce swollen tissue around the aching joint. Mix 6 drops of the oil with 1 tablespoon of carrier oil, and massage into the affected area. Repeat daily.

Asthma – asthma sufferers can benefit greatly from using eucalyptus oil to ease their symptoms. The aroma from the oil dilates blood vessels, thereby increasing oxygen supply to the lungs, which regulates breathing. Blend 5 drops of the oil with 1 teaspoon of carrier oil, and massage into the chest area.

Bites & Stings – eucalyptus oil contains excellent antiseptic qualities, protecting any insect bite or sting from becoming infected. Mix 2 drops with ½ teaspoon of coconut oil, and massage over the affected area. Repeat 2-3 times per day.

Bronchitis – eucalyptus oil's valuable expectorant properties make it a beneficial oil to use for treating bronchitis. It helps to clear mucus and reduce inflammation around the airways. Add 5 drops to a steam inhalation, and inhale the vapor deeply for 3-4 minutes. You can also mix 5 drops of the oil with 1 teaspoon of carrier oil, and massage into the chest area.

Colds & Flu – eucalyptus oil is perhaps best known for its action on the upper respiratory tract due to its natural decongestant action. Its antibacterial and anti-inflammatory properties also help to clear the viral infection and ease breathing by reducing inflammation of the nasal passageways. Add 4 drops to a steam inhalation, and breathe deeply for 3-4 minutes, taking a break if you need to. You can also mix 4 drops with 1 teaspoon of carrier oil, and massage into the chest area.

Cuts & Abrasions – mix 3 drops with ½ teaspoon of coconut oil, and massage over the affected area. Alternatively, add 1 drop to a cold compress and hold over the cut or wound for 5 minutes. Eucalyptus oil cleanses minor cuts and abrasions, and is effective in destroying any bacteria that may be present.

Cystitis – eucalyptus oil is useful for disorders of the urinary tract including cystitis as it helps to clear infection, reduce inflammation, and ease stinging or burning sensations. Add 4 drops to a cold compress, and hold over the affected area for 5 minutes. Alternatively, dilute 5 drops of the oil in 1 tablespoon of carrier oil, and add to a sitz bath. Sit for 20 minutes.

Diabetes – eucalyptus oil increases oxygen supply to the cells of the body through its ability to activate red blood cell functioning, thereby increasing blood circulation and lowering blood sugar levels, both of which benefit diabetes sufferers. After showering, massage a blend of 7 drops of eucalyptus oil with 2 tablespoons of carrier oil into the body. Repeat 3 times per week.

Ear Infections – mix 4 drops of eucalyptus oil with 1 teaspoon of carrier oil, and massage into the front and back of the ear. Never pour the formula inside the eardrum. Eucalyptus oil helps to fight an ear infection, reduce inflammation, and ease any pain and discomfort.

Fever – eucalyptus oil has a cooling effect on the body, and is therefore useful in reducing body temperature during fever. Diffuse 5 drops of the oil in your home to cool the air or, mix 8 drops with 2 tablespoons of carrier oil, and massage into the body. Repeat twice per day.

Gingivitis – eucalyptus oil's antibacterial and germicidal properties work at easing gingivitis by helping to kill the infection. It also possesses excellent anti-inflammatory properties, which help to reduce inflamed gums. Add 2 drops to a small amount of water, and use as a mouth rinse. Do not swallow.

Immune System – mix 5 drops with 1 teaspoon of carrier oil, and massage into the feet and heels. Eucalyptus oil acts as a tonic for the body, protecting it from illness by boosting and strengthening the immune system.

Jet Lag – place 3 drops of eucalyptus oil on a tissue, and inhale regularly. Alternatively, mix 5 drops with 1 teaspoon of carrier oil, and massage into the chest area. Eucalyptus oil has a refreshing, stimulating effect on the mind, helping to awaken the senses and keep the mind alert and focused.

Mental Clarity – eucalyptus oil refreshes and stimulates the brain, clearing mental exhaustion and fatigue. Diffuse 5 drops to clear any sluggishness from the air. You can also mix 6 drops with 1 teaspoon of carrier oil, and massage into the chest area, across the shoulders, and behind the neck. Another simple way to encourage mental alertness is to place 3 drops on a tissue, and inhale throughout the day.

Muscular Aches & Pains – massaging eucalyptus oil over sore muscles helps to relieve aches and pains as it contains strong analgesic and anti-inflammatory properties. Mix 5 drops with 1 tablespoon of carrier oil, and massage into the aching muscle. Alternatively, dilute 6 drops in 1 tablespoon of carrier oil, and add to a warm bath. Repeat daily.

Neuralgia – the pain associated with facial neuralgia can be treated using eucalyptus oil. Mix 3 drops with 1 teaspoon of coconut oil, and gently massage into the area of concern. Repeat daily.

Oily, Congested Skin – when used in steaming, eucalyptus oil can have a cleansing effect on congested, oily skin. Add 5 drops to a facial steamer, and allow 5 minutes for the vapor to penetrate the skin.

Shingles – the symptoms of shingles include pain, swelling, itching, and the risk of infection, all of which can be eased by massaging a blend of eucalyptus oil into the skin. Mix 7 drops with 2 tablespoons of the oil, and gently massage into the body. You can also dilute 5 drops in 1 tablespoon of carrier oil, and add to a warm bath.

Sinusitis – add 4 drops to a steam inhalation, and breathe deeply for 2-3 minutes. You can also diffuse 5 drops, or place 3 drops on a tissue, and inhale when you feel the need. The powerful decongestant properties found in eucalyptus oil ease the symptoms of sinusitis.

Sore Throat – eucalyptus oil helps to soothe a sore throat by easing any pain and reducing inflammation in that area. Add 4 drops of the oil to a small amount of water, and gargle for 40 seconds. Repeat 2-3 times per day. Do not swallow.

Fennel Oil

Fennel oil acts as a tonic for the digestive system, providing quick relief from hiccups, flatulence, nausea, vomiting, indigestion, and constipation. Its diuretic action speeds up the elimination of waste materials from the body, reduces water retention, and breaks up the fatty deposits under the surface of the skin that result in cellulite. As a tonic for the female reproductive system, fennel oil helps to regularize menstruation, relieve menstrual cramps and PMS, and ease menopausal symptoms.

Properties: antimicrobial, antiseptic, antispasmodic, carminative, depurative, diuretic, emmenagogue, expectorant, galactogogue, laxative, stomachic, tonic.

Ways to Use Fennel Essential Oil

Cellulite – fennel oil helps to reduce the appearance of cellulite due to its diuretic and detoxifying properties. Blend 5 drops with 1 tablespoon of coconut oil, and firmly massage into areas of concern. Repeat daily.

Constipation – fennel oil is an effective laxative and can help with cases of constipation. Mix 4 drops with 1 teaspoon of carrier oil, and massage into the abdomen. Repeat twice per day.

Detox – fennel oil has strong detoxifying properties, helping to reduce water retention and break up the accumulation of toxic wastes, eliminating them from the body. Mix 4 drops with 1 teaspoon of carrier oil, and massage into the soles of the feet. You can also dilute 6 drops in 1 tablespoon of carrier oil, and add to a warm Epsom salt bath.

Digestion – fennel oil acts as a tonic for the digestive system as a whole, keeping the stomach and intestines in good working order. Mix 4 drops with 1 teaspoon of carrier oil, and massage into the abdomen, or massage into both feet. Repeat daily.

Fluid Retention – fennel oil's strong diuretic properties increase urination, which in turn, helps to reduce water retention in the body's tissues. Dilute 7 drops in 1 tablespoon of carrier oil, and add to a warm Epsom salt bath.

Heartburn – mix 5 drops with 1 teaspoon of carrier oil, and massage into the chest and abdominal region. Massage using circular, clockwise movements. Fennel oil helps to ease acid reflux which causes indigestion.

Irregular Periods – fennel oil has an excellent effect on the female reproductive system, helping to regulate the menstrual cycle. Mix 4 drops of the oil with 1 teaspoon of carrier oil, and massage into the lower abdomen. Repeat daily until the problem disappears.

Kidney Stones – fennel oil's excellent detoxifying capabilities help to prevent the accumulation of kidney stones and have a toning effect on the kidneys. Mix 4 drops with 1 teaspoon of carrier oil, and massage into the feet. You can also dilute 6 drops with 1 tablespoon of carrier oil, and add to a warm bath.

Mature Skin – mix 3 drops with 1 teaspoon of fennel oil, and massage into the face and neck. Fennel oil helps to maintain muscle tone in the face and improve skin elasticity. Repeat 2-3 times per week.

Menopause – fennel oil stimulates the production of estrogen by the adrenal glands after the ovaries have ceased functioning, which can delay the onset of menopause, or reduce the unpleasant symptoms during menopause. Dilute 6 drops in 1 tablespoon of carrier oil, and add to a warm bath. Alternatively, you can mix 7 drops with 2 tablespoons of carrier oil, and use as a massage oil for the body. Repeat 3-4 times per week.

Menstrual Cramps – mix 4 drops of fennel oil with 1 teaspoon of carrier oil, and massage into the abdomen. You can also add 3 drops to a hot compress, and drape over the lower abdomen for 10 minutes at a time. Repeat twice per day. Fennel oil eases uterine spasms that cause the cramps.

Obesity – fennel oil is useful for treating obesity as it helps to suppress the appetite while, at the same time, ridding the body of toxic waste and water retention. Mix 4 drops with 1 teaspoon of carrier oil, and massage into the soles of the feet. You can also drink fennel tea which can be purchased from most health shops.

PMS – fennel oil helps to reduce the symptoms of PMS by regulating hormones and easing mood swings, nausea, and irritability. Diffuse 5 drops, or add a blend of 6 drops with 1 tablespoon of carrier oil to a warm bath.

Rheumatism & Arthritis – mix 4 drops of fennel oil, and massage into the affected area, paying particular attention to painful joints. Fennel oil helps to reduce inflammation of the joints by preventing and reducing the build up of toxins that accumulate around the joint area.

Urinary Tract Infections – fennel oil acts as a tonic for the urinary tract, cleansing the kidneys to help protect against infections. Mix 4 drops with 1 teaspoon of carrier oil, and massage into the mid to lower back. You can also massage the formula into the soles of the feet.

Frankincense Oil

Great for both mature and oily skin, frankincense oil helps to improve skin tone, smooth and soften wrinkles, and balance sebum levels. It is also effective in comforting and calming the mind, reducing the appearance of scars and stretch marks, and easing respiratory disorders such as asthma and bronchitis.

Properties: anticatarrhal, antiseptic, antitussive, astringent, calming, carminative, cicatrisant, cytopylactic, diuretic, emmenagogue, expectorant, rubefacient, sedative, tonic, uterine, vulnerary.

Ways to Use Frankincense Essential Oil

Asthma – frankincense oil helps to promote deep, slow breathing, thereby lessening the chances of an asthma attack. Diffuse 5 drops, or place 2 drops on a tissue, and inhale regularly. You can also mix 5 drops with 1 teaspoon of carrier oil, and massage into the chest area.

Bad Breath – frankincense oil has strong antiseptic qualities and can act as a preventative measure against bad breath. Add 2 drops of the oil to a small glass of water, and use as a mouth wash. Do not swallow.

Breast Health – mix 4 drops of frankincense oil with 1 teaspoon of carrier oil, and massage thoroughly into the breasts. Frankincense oil promotes healthy breast tissue and reduces breast inflammation.

Brittle Nails – mix 2 drops with ½ teaspoon of coconut oil, and massage into each nail and around the cuticle to strengthen weak nails.

Bronchitis – frankincense oil helps to soothe the respiratory tract, and clear congestion from the lungs. It also eases shortness of breath and calms the symptoms of bronchitis. Diffuse 5 drops of the oil, or place 2 drops on a tissue, and inhale regularly. Alternatively, mix 4 drops with 1 teaspoon of carrier oil, and massage into the chest.

Coughing – add 3 drops of frankincense oil to a steam inhalation, and inhale for 2-3 minutes, taking a break if necessary. Frankincense oil soothes a cough and helps to expel any mucus in the respiratory tract. Repeat twice per day until symptoms clear.

Cystitis – dilute 5 drops in 1 tablespoon of carrier oil, and add to a sitz bath. Sit for 20 minutes. Frankincense oil eases the symptoms of cystitis including inflammation, stinging, and any emotional stress that may be encountered.

Dysmenhorrhea (Heavy Menstrual Bleeding) – mix 5 drops with 1 tablespoon of carrier oil, and massage into the abdomen. Frankincense oil helps to tone the uterus and relieve heavy menstrual bleeding.

Emotional Balance – diffusing frankincense oil helps to calm the emotions, breaking links with the past that may otherwise lead to physical illness. Diffuse 5 drops in the home.

Focus & Concentration – frankincense oil revitalizes the mind, helping to reduce internal chatter. Diffuse 5 drops, or place 2 drops on a tissue, and inhale regularly.

Immune System – blend 8 drops of frankincense oil with 2 tablespoons of carrier oil, and massage into the body. Alternatively, dilute 6 drops in 1 tablespoon of carrier oil, and add to a bath of warm water. Frankincense oil is a great immune system booster as it helps to clear internal and external wounds, fight infection, and kill any germs.

Mental or Physical Exhaustion – frankincense oil soothes and uplifts the mind, which in turn revitalizes the physical body. Diffuse 5 drops of the oil, or dilute 6 drops in 1 tablespoon of carrier oil, and add to a warm bath. Alternatively, mix 5 drops with 1 teaspoon of carrier oil, and massage into the feet.

Oily Skin – frankincense oil's astringent properties help to balance oily skin, cleanse and tighten open pores, and help maintain skin elasticity. Mix 4 drops with 1 teaspoon of coconut oil, and massage into the face and neck. Leave the oils to absorb into the skin. Repeat twice daily.

Scarring – mix 2 drops of frankincense oil with ½ teaspoon of coconut oil, and gently massage into scar tissue. Repeat 2-3 times per day. Frankincense oil promotes the growth of new skin cells, which grow over scar tissue to eventually smooth the skin. Repeat twice per day.

Stress or Tension – diffuse 5 drops of frankincense oil to create a place of peace and relaxation. You can also dilute 6 drops in 1 tablespoon of carrier oil, and add to a warm bath. Frankincense oil promotes deep breathing and relaxation, making you feel more at ease.

Stretch Marks – frankincense oil helps to tone a slack looking skin and support the development of new skin cells, helping to significantly reduce or prevent stretch marks when used regularly. Mix 5 drops of the oil with 1 tablespoon of coconut oil, and massage into the affected area. Repeat twice per day.

Sun Spots – regular application of frankincense oil over sun pots can fade their appearance significantly and heal the skin. Mix 1 drop of the oil with ¼ teaspoon of coconut oil, and massage over the sun spot twice per day.

Uterine Cyst – frankincense oil acts as an overall uterine tonic as it regulates the production of estrogen. It therefore helps to maintain a healthy uterus and reduce the risk of cyst formation. Mix 4 drops with 1 teaspoon of carrier oil, and massage into the abdomen in a clockwise direction.

Wounds & Ulcers – frankincense oil speeds up the recovery of any wounds, cuts or ulcers, both internally and externally. It also protects from infection. Mix 2 drops of the oil with ½ teaspoon of coconut oil, and massage over the wound 2-3 times per day.

Wrinkles – known for its wonderful skin rejuvenating properties, frankincense oil helps to prevent or reduce wrinkles and tone the skin. Mix 4 drops with 1 teaspoon of coconut oil, and massage into the face and neck. Repeat daily, morning and night.

Geranium Oil

A wonderful all-round oil for the skin; geranium revitalizes skin cells, helps to control sebum production in oily skin, helps to keep the skin supple, and rejuvenates pale, dull skin. It also helps to ease menstrual problems and improve circulation.

Properties: antidepressant, anti-inflammatory, antiseptic, astringent, balancing, cicatrisant, cytophylactic, diuretic, deodorant, hemostatic, stimulant, tonic, uplifting, vermifuge, vulnerary.

Ways to Use Geranium Essential Oil

Broken Capillaries – geranium oil has excellent astringent properties resulting in the contraction of blood vessels, which over time, will lessen the appearance of dilated or broken capillaries. Mix 2 drops with ½ teaspoon of coconut oil, and very gently apply over the affected area. Do not massage into the skin. Repeat daily.

Cellulite – geranium oil stimulates the lymphatic system, helping to diminish water retention and eliminate toxins, which reduce the appearance of cellulite over time. Mix 6 drops of the oil with 1 tablespoon of coconut oil, and firmly massage into affected areas. Alternatively, dilute 6 drops in 1 tablespoon of carrier oil, and add to a warm bath (a cup of Epsom salts will help the elimination of toxins). Repeat 3-4 times per week.

Chilblains – mix 5 drops with 1 tablespoon of carrier oil, and gently massage the affected area. Always massage in the direction of the heart. Geranium oil stimulates a sluggish circulation, therefore improving blood flow.

Deodorant – geranium oil has a minty, fresh fragrance that creates a beautiful natural deodorant. It also contains antibacterial properties, which help to kill the germs that create body odor. Mix 15 drops of the oil with ¼ cup of baking soda, and rub onto the armpits.

Detox – dilute 6 drops in 1 tablespoon of carrier oil, and add to a warm Epsom salt bath. Alternatively, mix 4 drops of the oil with 1 teaspoon of carrier oil, and massage into the feet. The diuretic properties of geranium oil increase the quantity and frequency of urination, resulting in increased elimination of toxins from the body.

Digestion – geranium oil facilitates improved digestion of ingested foods through increased urination. Mix 5 drops of the oil with 1 tablespoon of carrier oil, and massage into the abdomen in a clockwise direction.

Dysmenorrhea (heavy menstrual bleeding) – mix 5 drops with 1 tablespoon of carrier oil, and massage into the abdomen. Geranium oil balances the hormones thus regulating heavy periods.

Emotional Balance – geranium oil is perhaps best known for its balancing properties. Diffusing 6 drops of this beautiful oil will help to alleviate mood swings, restore calm to the mind and body, and promote a general feeling of well-being.

Flatulence – geranium oil promotes increased urination due to its diuretic properties, and as a result, prevents the formation of gas in the intestines. Mix 5 drops with 1 tablespoon, and massage into the abdomen in a clockwise direction.

Gums & Teeth – add 1 drop of geranium oil to 1 teaspoon of aloe vera gel, and rub into the gums. Leave for 10 minutes, do not swallow. Add 2 drops to a small glass of water, and use as a mouth rinse, do not swallow. The astringent properties in geranium oil help the gums to contract and tighten, lessening the chance of tooth loss.

Impetigo – geranium oil is an excellent overall tonic for the body, and helps to speed up the healing process of the skin. Its antibacterial action also prevents the spread of this skin disorder. Mix 1 drop with ¼ teaspoon of coconut oil, and apply over the infection using a cotton bud. Repeat 2-3 times per day using a clean cotton bud each time.

Insomnia – geranium oil helps to balance the nervous system and calms an overactive mind, which can often interfere with a peaceful night's sleep. Place 2 drops on the pillow before bedtime, or diffuse 3 drops 1 hour before bedtime.

Kidney Stones – geranium oil has a tonic effect on the kidneys, therefore making it a beneficial treatment for kidney stones. Dilute 6 drops in 1 tablespoon of carrier oil, and add to a warm bath. Alternatively, blend 4 drops with 1 tablespoon of carrier oil, and massage into the soles of the feet.

Menopause – geranium oil helps to balance the secretion of female hormones by regulating the adrenal cortex. Dilute 6 drops in 1 tablespoon of carrier oil, and add to a warm bath. Alternatively, mix 4 drops with 1 teaspoon of carrier oil, and massage into the feet. To dispel negative emotions associated with menopause, diffuse 5 drops of the oil, and allow the fresh scent to fill the room.

Oily Skin – geranium oil helps to clear congested skin and balance oil production. Mix 4 drops with 1 teaspoon of coconut oil, and massage into the face and neck. Alternatively, add 3 drops to your moisturizer each morning, and carry out your skincare regime as normal.

PMS – because geranium oil is a powerful regulator in hormone secretion, it is a perfect oil to use when treating symptoms linked to PMS. It helps to lessen anxiety, alleviate mood swings, reduce irritation and anger, and promote feelings of euphoria. Mix 5 drops with 1 tablespoon of carrier oil, and massage into the abdomen. You can also diffuse 5 drops of the oil.

Poor Circulation – geranium oil helps to enlarge capillaries, thus helping to improve blood circulation. Mix 8 drops with 2 tablespoons of carrier oil, and massage the body. Also, dilute 6 drops in 1 tablespoon of carrier oil, and add to a warm bath.

Scarring – whether the scars are caused by acne, surgery, or chicken pox, geranium oil has excellent cicatrisant properties making scars fade over time with regular use. Mix 2 drops of the oil with ½ teaspoon of coconut oil, and gently massage directly over the scar. Repeat twice per day.

Stress & Anxiety – geranium oil helps to balance the nervous system, restoring calm to the body in times of stress. Place 2 drops of the oil on a tissue, and inhale regularly, or diffuse 5 drops to dispel any negative energy in the room. You can also add 15 drops to a 300ml spray bottle filled with filtered water, and spray over the upper body when needed. Shake well before use.

Wrinkles – geranium oil promotes skin cell regeneration and tightens sagging muscles and skin. Mix 5 drops with 1 teaspoon of coconut oil, and massage into the face and neck. Repeat twice per day.

Ginger Oil

Ginger oil is very often used to treat motion sickness and nausea. It eases digestive disorders such as indigestion, diarrhea, and vomiting, and also helps to clear a congested respiratory tract. It has a strong warming action on the body, which helps to ease arthritic and rheumatic pain. It is an excellent oil to use on muscles post exercise to help alleviate any tightness.

Properties: analgesic, antiseptic, antispasmodic, carminative, expectorant, febrifuge, laxative, rubefacient, stimulant, stomachic, sudorific, tonic, warming.

Ways to Use Ginger Essential Oil

Arthritis – ginger oil's warming action, together with its analgesic properties, help to soothe painful joints, relieving the symptoms of arthritis. Mix 3 drops with 1 teaspoon of carrier oil, and massage over the area of concern.

Bruises – ginger oil's ability to improve blood circulation helps to speed up the healing of bruises. Mix 2 drops with ½ teaspoon of coconut oil, and gently massage over the bruise 2-3 times per day.

Chilblains – ginger oil helps to warm chills and increase blood circulation. Dilute 4 drops in 1 tablespoon of carrier oil, and add to a warm bath. You can also massage into the feet using a blend of 3 drops of ginger oil with 1 teaspoon of carrier oil.

Colds & Flu – ginger oil eases cold and flu symptoms such as runny nose, sore throat, and a build up of phlegm in the chest area. Add 3 drops to a steam inhalation, or dilute 4 drops in 1 tablespoon of carrier oil, and add to a warm bath. Soak for 10 minutes.

Confidence – ginger oil opens the heart and instils feelings of self confidence and self esteem. Diffuse 3 drops, or apply 2 drops to a tissue, and inhale regularly.

Digestion – ginger oil stimulates the secretion of digestive juices, helping to maintain a healthy digestive tract. Mix 3 drops with 1 teaspoon of carrier oil, and massage into the abdomen.

Fatigue – ginger oil has a stimulating effect on body and mind, invigorating the senses and increasing vitality and energy. Mix 3 drops with 1 teaspoon of carrier oil, and massage into the feet, or simply diffuse 3 drops in your home to clear sluggish energy.

Fever – diffuse 3 drops in your home, or add 3 drops to a large bowl of cold water and pat down the body. Ginger oil encourages sweating, which in turn helps to cool the body down and ultimately break the fever.

Flatulence – ginger oil helps to eliminate a build up of gas from the body. Mix 3 drops with 1 teaspoon of carrier oil, and massage into the lower abdomen.

Menstrual Cramps – ginger oil relieves menstrual cramps by easing spasms in the uterus. Mix 3 drops of the oil with 1 teaspoon of carrier oil, and massage into the lower abdomen.

Motion Sickness – perhaps best known for its effect on motion sickness, ginger oil helps to calm an upset stomach and reduce dizziness and/or nausea. Mix 2 drops with ½ teaspoon of carrier oil, and massage behind and just under the ears. Alternatively, place 2 drops on a tissue, and inhale regularly when travelling.

Muscular Aches & Pains – ginger oil provides relief from aching muscles and eases spasm in the muscles. Add 4 drops to a warm compress, and drape over sore muscles for 10-20 minutes. Alternatively, mix 4 drops with 1 tablespoon of carrier oil, and massage into the area of concern. You can also dilute 4 drops in 1 tablespoon of carrier oil, and add to a warm bath.

Sinusitis – add 3 drops to a steam inhalation, or place 2 drops on a tissue, and inhale regularly throughout the day. Ginger oil helps to clear mucus from the nasal passageways.

Sore Throat – add 2 drops to a small amount of water, and gargle for 20-30 seconds. Do not swallow. Ginger oil helps to reduce an inflamed throat and ease any pain or discomfort.

Varicose Veins – ginger oil stimulates the circulation, helping to speed up sluggish blood circulation around the body. Mix 3 drops with 1 teaspoon of carrier oil, and gently massage over the entire limb. Do not massage directly over varicose veins. Always massage upwards in the direction of the heart.

Grapefruit Oil

An excellent mentally uplifting and refreshing oil, grapefruit helps to ease a stressed body and mind. It has fantastic astringent properties making it a great choice for oily, dull skin, and acne. Grapefruit oil is also well known for its treatment of cellulite as it helps to dissolve fat deposits and reduce fluid retention.

Properties: antidepressant, antiseptic, astringent, depurative, diuretic, disinfectant, stimulant, tonic, uplifting.

Ways to Use Grapefruit Essential Oil

Acne – grapefruit oil possesses potent antiseptic, astringent, and bactericidal properties, making it an ideal oil to use in the treatment of acne. Mix 5 drops of the oil with 1 teaspoon of coconut oil, and massage into the face and neck. You can also add 3 drops to ½ teaspoon of aloe vera gel, and apply directly over pimples. Repeat twice per day after cleansing, and leave the oils to absorb into the skin.

Arthritis – grapefruit oil's diuretic properties help to eliminate waste materials such as uric acid, which is a common cause of arthritis. Dilute 6 drops of the oil with 1 tablespoon of carrier oil, and add to a warm bath. Alternatively, blend 8 drops with 2 tablespoons of carrier oil, and massage into the body, paying particular attention to the major joints of the body such as the ankles, wrists, hips, and shoulders. Repeat daily.

Cellulite – mix 6 drops of grapefruit oil with 1 tablespoon of coconut oil, and firmly massage into affected areas. For larger areas, mix 8 drops of the oil with 2 tablespoons of carrier oil. Grapefruit oil encourages the elimination of toxins that accumulate in the cells of the body, creating cellulite. Repeat every day for excellent results.

Depression – grapefruit oil contains powerful stimulating and uplifting properties, helping to provoke positive feelings of hope, happiness, and peacefulness. Diffuse 6 drops of the oil in the home, or place 2 drops on a tissue, and inhale regularly.

Digestion – mix 5 drops of grapefruit oil with 1 teaspoon of carrier oil, and massage into the abdomen using circular, clockwise movements. Grapefruit oil stimulates the secretion of gastric juices and bile in the stomach, aiding efficient digestion.

Fluid Retention – grapefruit oil's strong diuretic properties help to rid the body of excess fluids by promoting urination. Dilute 6 drops in 1 tablespoon of carrier oil, and add to a warm bath. Alternatively, mix 6 drops with 1 teaspoon of carrier oil, and massage into the soles of the feet. Repeat every day until symptoms clear.

Healthy Hair – grapefruit oil promotes healthy hair. By adding 5 drops to 1 ounce of shampoo it can strengthen the hair follicle and leave your hair with a beautiful shine. You can also treat dandruff by massaging 5 drops of the oil and 1 teaspoon of olive oil into the scalp.

Immune System – diffuse 5 drops in your home, or mix 5 drops with 1 teaspoon of carrier oil, and massage into the soles of the feet. You can also dilute 6 drops in 1 tablespoon of carrier oil, and add to a warm bath. Grapefruit oil is rich in vitamin C and antioxidants, which helps to keep the immune system strong and protected against colds and flu. Repeat regularly especially during the winter months.

Jet Lag – mix 5 drops of grapefruit oil with 1 teaspoon of carrier oil, and massage into the chest, and front and back of the neck. You can also place 3 drops on a tissue, and inhale regularly. Grapefruit oil invigorates and revitalizes a tired body and mind.

Kidney Function – grapefruit oil promotes increased urination due to its diuretic properties, which maintains the proper functioning of the kidneys. Mix 5 drops of the oil with 1 teaspoon of carrier oil, and massage into the soles of the feet. Also, blend 6 drops with 1 tablespoon of carrier oil, and add to a warm bath.

Lethargy – grapefruit oil is a great 'pick me up' oil as it stimulates the nervous system, reviving both body and mind. Diffuse 6 drops in the home, or mix 6 drops with 1 teaspoon of carrier oil, and massage into the feet. Leave the oils to absorb into the skin.

Migraines – migraines can be treated using grapefruit oil, particularly where they are stress related. Diffuse 3 drops, or mix 2 drops with 1 teaspoon of carrier oil, and massage into the forehead and temples.

Obesity – grapefruit oil can help to decrease appetite, curb any cravings you may have, and prevent binge eating. Diffuse 6 drops in your home, or place 3 drops on a tissue, and inhale each time you feel any weakness towards food.

Oily Skin – the astringent and antiseptic properties of grapefruit oil make it perfect for use on oily skin. It helps to cleanse congested skin, tighten open pores, and improve skin elasticity. Mix 4 drops with 1 teaspoon of coconut oil, and massage into the face and neck. Leave the oils to absorb into the skin. Repeat daily.

PMS – diffuse 5 drops of the oil, or mix 5 drops with 1 teaspoon of carrier oil, and massage into the feet. Grapefruit oil promotes positive feelings by stimulating certain neurotransmitters in the brain. It addresses issues of self image, frustration and anger.

Helichrysum Oil

Excellent for treating various skin disorders, helichrysum oil fights bacterial infections, reduces inflammation, and promotes healing. It stimulates digestion and is recommended for irritable bowel syndrome, indigestion, and intestinal cramps. It also relieves muscular spasms, menstrual cramps, and heart palpitations, and also eases the pain of arthritis, rheumatism, sciatica, backache, and muscle ache.

Properties: antibacterial, anti-inflammatory, antimicrobial, antioxidant, antiseptic, antispasmodic, astringent, cholagogue, cicatrisant, diuretic, expectorant, hepatic, mucolytic, stimulant.

Ways to Use Helichrysum Essential Oil

Arthritis – because of its anti-inflammatory and analgesic properties, helichrysum oil helps to relieve the pain and swelling that accompanies arthritis. Mix 4 drops with 1 teaspoon of carrier oil, and massage into the area of concern.

Athlete's Foot – helichrysum oil's fungicidal capabilities help to destroy the fungal bacteria which cause athlete's foot. It also helps to hinder the spread of the infection. Mix 3 drops of the oil with 1 teaspoon of coconut oil, and massage into the feet and toes. Make sure your feet have been cleaned thoroughly.

Bruises – helichrysum oil helps to speed up the healing of bruises. Mix 2 drops with ½ teaspoon of carrier oil, and gently massage over the area of concern twice per day.

Cold Sores – mix 1 drop of helichrysum oil with 1 drop of coconut oil, and apply to the cold sore directly using a cotton bud. Helichrysum oil helps to kill the viral infection and speed up the healing process.

Coughing – helichrysum oil helps to clear excess mucus from the respiratory tract, providing relief from coughing. Mix 3 drops with 1 teaspoon of carrier oil, and massage into the chest area. You can also add 2 drops to a steam inhalation, and inhale deeply for 3-4 minutes. Repeat twice per day until symptoms clear.

Detox – helichrysum oil helps to cleanse the liver, and also promotes increased urination due to its diuretic properties, which in turn speeds up the elimination of wastes and toxins from the blood. Dilute 4 drops in 1 teaspoon of carrier oil, and add to a warm Epsom salt bath. Alternatively, mix 3 drops with 1 teaspoon of carrier oil, and massage into the feet.

Fever – dilute 5 drops in 1 tablespoon of carrier oil, and add to a warm bath. Soak for 20 minutes. Alternatively, mix 3 drops with 1 teaspoon of carrier oil, and massage into the feet. Repeat the foot massage twice per day. Helichrysum oil helps to reduce the fever and clear the infection.

Hemmorrhaging – helichrysum oil helps to prevent blood clots by thinning the blood. It also prevents hemorrhaging. Mix 3 drops with 1 teaspoon of carrier oil, and massage into the soles of the feet.

High Blood Pressure – an increase in the quantity and frequency of urination is brought about by helichrysum oil's excellent diuretic properties. This increase helps to rid the body of wastes, reducing cholesterol levels and lowering high blood pressure. Dilute 4 drops in 1 tablespoon of carrier oil, and add to a warm bath. Alternatively, mix 3 drops with 1 teaspoon of carrier oil, and massage into the feet.

Immune System – helichrysum oil possesses potent antimicrobial, antioxidant, antibacterial, anti-inflammatory, and antispasmodic properties, which collectively help to keep the immune system healthy, strong, and infection free. Mix 5 drops with 2 tablespoons of carrier oil, and massage into the body. Alternatively, you can also dilute 5 drops with 1 tablespoon of carrier oil, and add to a warm bath, or mix 3 drops with 1 teaspoon of carrier oil, and massage into the feet

Indigestion – mix 4 drops with 1 teaspoon of carrier oil, and massage into the abdomen in a clockwise direction. Helichrysum oil promotes the secretion of bile in the stomach and helps to neutralize stomach acids, which cause heartburn or indigestion.

Liver Function – helichrysum oil acts as a tonic for the liver, ensuring proper function by cleansing and detoxifying, therefore keeping the liver healthy and strong. Mix 3 drops with 1 teaspoon of carrier oil, and massage into the upper left abdominal region. Alternatively, you can massage the formula into the soles of the feet.

Mature Skin – helichrysum oil promotes the removal of dead skin cells from the surface of the skin and stimulates the production of new cells, helping to rejuvenate older skin. Mix 4 drops of the oil with 1 teaspoon of coconut oil, and massage into the face and neck. You can also add 2 drops to your moistuizer each day, and moisturize as normal. Repeat daily.

Muscular Aches & Pains – mix 5 drops with 1 tablespoon of carrier oil, and massage into sore muscles. Helichrysum oil soothes aching muscles, helping to alleviate pain and reduce any inflammation that may be present.

Nasal Congestion – helichrysum oil loosens the build up of phlegm and congestion from the air passageways, easing a blocked nose. Add 3 drops to a steam inhalation, and inhale deeply for 3-4 minutes. You can also mix 3 drops with 1 teaspoon of carrier oil, and massage into the upper chest.

Rheumatism – helichrysum oil eases the neuralgia with rheumatism, and therefore helps to reduce pain in the joints. Mix 4 drops with 1 teaspoon of carrier oil, and massage into the joints. You may need to increase the formula if you experience pain in more than 1 area – mix 5 drops with 1 tablespoon of carrier oil.

Scar Tissue – helichrysum oil is perhaps best known for its ability to heal scar tissue, whether new or old. It has excellent cell regenerating properties, thus helping the scar tissue to repair itself. Mix 3 drops with ½ teaspoon of coconut oil, and massage over the scar twice per day.

Splenic Tonic – with splenic properties, helichrysum oil helps to keep the spleen healthy, strong, and infection free. Mix 3 drops with 1 teaspoon of coconut oil, and massage into both feet.

Sprains & Strains – whether related to muscle or bone, helichrysum oil eases pain and helps to reduce swollen tissue or muscles. Mix 3 drops with 1 teaspoon of carrier oil, and very gently massage into the affected area. Repeat twice daily until symptoms ease.

Wrinkles – mix 4 drops of helichrysum oil with 1 teaspoon of coconut oil, and massage into the face and neck. Helichrysum oil helps to diminish fine lines and wrinkles, and when used regularly, it helps delay the formation of wrinkles.

Hyssop Oil

Hyssop oil can be used to heal wounds and bruising on the skin. It contains expectorant, antibacterial, and antiviral properties that make it a valuable treatment for respiratory disorders such as bronchitis, influenza, asthma, coughing, colds, and laryngitis. Bloating and water retention are reduced with the use of hyssop oil. It also helps to ease stress and anxiety, and alleviate fatigue.

Properties: antiseptic, antirheumatic, antispasmodic, astringent, carminative, cicatrisant, digestive, diuretic, emmenagogue, expectorant, febrifuge, hypertensive, nervine, stimulant, sudorific, tonic, vulnerary.

Ways to Use Hyssop Essential Oil

Bronchitis – mix 2 drops with 1 teaspoon of carrier oil, and massage into the chest area. Hyssop oil is effective in relieving congestion and calming persistent coughing.

Bruising – hyssop oil is an effective treatment for bruising, helping to heal the area at a faster rate. Add 1-2 drops on a cold compress, and place over the area of concern.

Colds & Flu – hyssop oil is very effective at fluidifying mucus so it can be expelled more easily. Add 2 drops to a steam inhalation, or mix 2 drops with 1 teaspoon of carrier oil, and massage into the chest area.

Coughing – hyssop oil helps to clear mucus that obstructs the airways causing persistent, exhausting coughing. Add 3 drops to a steam inhalation, or mix 4 drops with 1 teaspoon of carrier oil, and massage into the chest.

Creativity – hyssop oil invigorates and uplifts the mind, which stimulates creativity and focus. Diffuse 2 drops to dispel a sluggish energy.

Digestion – mix 2 drops with 1 teaspoon of carrier oil, and massage into the abdomen in a clockwise direction. Hyssop oil acts as a tonic for the digestive system as it stimulates digestion and warms the stomach.

Irregular Menstruation – hyssop oil encourages menstruation and can help to normalize obstructed, irregular periods. Mix 2 drops with 1 teaspoon of carrier oil, and massage into the lower abdomen in a clockwise direction.

Low Blood Pressure – hyssop oil has a normalizing effect on the circulation and helps to raise low blood sugar. Mix 2 drops with 1 teaspoon of carrier oil, and massage over the heart area.

Rheumatism – hyssop oil helps to ease the symptoms of rheumatism by promoting and maintaining circulation. Mix 2 drops with 1 teaspoon of carrier oil, and massage into the affected area.

Sore Throat – hyssop oil helps to relieve a painful, inflamed throat by gargling a small amount of water with 1 drop of the oil. Do not swallow.

Jasmine Oil

A fantastic oil for use on mature skin, jasmine oil helps to improve skin elasticity and encourage cell renewal. It is useful for treating stretch marks and scars, easing muscle aches and pains, and balancing hormones during PMS and menopause. It is also an uplifting, euphoric oil, helping to improve self confidence, calm nerves, and induce feelings of optimism.

Properties: antidepressant, antiseptic, antispasmodic, aphrodisiac, galactogogue, relaxing, sedative, uterine.

Ways to Use Jasmine Essential Oil

Aphrodisiac – jasmine oil is a valued aphrodisiac often used to promote sexual feelings and reduce male impotency or rigidity. Diffuse 4 drops in the bedroom, or mix 2 drops with ½ teaspoon of carrier oil, and massage over the heart center.

Breathing – mix 3 drops with 1 teaspoon of carrier oil, and massage into the chest area. Alternatively, place 2 drops on a tissue, and inhale regularly throughout the day. Jasmine oil helps to ease breathing difficulties by clearing any congestion in the respiratory tract.

Childbirth – mix 2 drops with 1 teaspoon of carrier oil, and massage into the lower abdomen, or massage into the soles of the feet. Jasmine oil helps to strengthen uterine contractions, therefore shortening the delivery time. It also helps to reduce labor pains.

Colds & Flu – when added to a steam inhalation, jasmine oil can help reduce infections that cause colds or flu, and therefore speed up the healing process. Add 3 drops to a steam inhalation, and breathe deeply for 3-4 minutes. Repeat daily until symptoms disappear.

Confidence – diffuse 3 drops of jasmine oil to improve self confidence and ease feelings of shyness. You can also blend 2 drops with ½ teaspoon of carrier oil, and massage over the heart area.

Contentment – jasmine oil helps to bring about feelings of contentment and happiness. Add 8 drops to a 300ml spray bottle filled with filtered water, and spray around the upper body when needed. Shake well before use. You can also diffuse 3 drops, or mix 2 drops with ½ teaspoon of carrier oil, and massage over the heart area.

Coughing – jasmine oil helps to clear out the build up of phlegm from the respiratory tract, clearing air passageways and relieving cough symptoms. Add 2 drops to a steam inhalation, and inhale deeply for 3-4 minutes. Alternatively, mix 3 drops with 1 teaspoon of carrier oil, and massage into the chest area.

Depression – jasmine oil has an uplifting effect on the mind, possessing potent antidepressant properties. It helps to instil feelings of optimism and hope to an otherwise negative mind. Diffuse 3 drops of jasmine oil in your home, or blend 2 drops with 1 teaspoon of carrier oil, and massage into the back of the neck and across the shoulders.

Dry Skin – mix 2 drops of jasmine oil with 1 teaspoon of coconut oil, and massage into the face, paying particular attention to any dry patches of skin. Jasmine oil helps to soothe and hydrate dry skin.

Eczema – jasmine oil relieves itching and inflammation associated with eczema and also helps to soothe dry patches of skin. Mix 2 drops with 1 teaspoon of coconut oil, and massage over the area of concern.

Emotional Imbalance – jasmine oil works on an emotional level, helping to calm frayed nerves and rectify emotional imbalance. Blend 3 drops of the oil with 1 teaspoon of carrier oil, and massage into the back of the neck and across the shoulders. You can also massage into the feet.

Insomnia – jasmine oil acts as a potent tranquilizer for the nervous system, instilling feelings of warmth and calm to promote a good night's sleep. Place 2 drops on your pillow before bedtime, or diffuse 3 drops in the bedroom.

Lactation – jasmine oil increases the secretion of breast milk during lactation, and also acts as a general tonic for breast tissue. Mix 2 drops with 1 teaspoon of carrier oil, and massage into the breasts.

Mature Skin – mix 3 drops with 1 teaspoon of coconut oil, and massage into the face and neck. Jasmine oil increases skin elasticity and promotes a toned skin. Repeat daily.

Menopause – jasmine oil helps to balance the emotions, therefore easing menopausal symptoms such as low energy, hot flashes, mood swings, and anxiety. Blend 3 drops with 1 teaspoon of carrier oil, and massage into the soles of the feet. Alternatively, add 10 drops to a 300ml spray bottle filled with filtered water, and spray around the upper body when you feel the onset of any of the above symptoms.

Menstrual Cramps – mix 3 drops with 1 teaspoon of carrier oil, and massage into the abdomen. Jasmine oil helps to relieve uterine spasms that cause painful period cramps.

Nervous Anxiety – jasmine oil has an uplifting effect, while at the same time, promoting calm and balance to the nervous system. Mix 3 drops of the oil with 1 teaspoon of carrier oil, and massage into the soles of the feet. You can also diffuse 3 drops to clear nervous tension from the air.

PMS – jasmine oil is effective in balancing the hormones, therefore alleviating mood swings, nervous anxiety, fatigue, and feelings of irritation. Diffuse 4 drops to clear negative energy, or mix 3 drops with 1 teaspoon of carrier oil, and massage into the feet.

Scar Tissue – mix 2 drops of jasmine oil with ½ teaspoon of coconut oil, and gently massage over scar tissue. Jasmine oil encourages the renewal of skin cells, helping to heal scar tissue over time. Repeat daily.

Stretch Marks – due to jasmine oil's cell regenerating properties, the appearance of stretch marks can be significantly reduced. When used regularly, jasmine oil helps to prevent stretch marks from forming. Mix 4 drops with 1 teaspoon of coconut oil, and massage into the area of concern.

Juniper Oil

Well known for its detoxifying and cleansing properties, juniper oil helps with fluid retention, cellulite, and acne. It helps to clear and stimulate the mind, as well as easing joint aches and pains. It is also a great tonic for the skin, relieving symptoms of dermatitis, eczema, and psoriasis.

Properties: antiseptic, antirheumatic, antispasmodic, astringent, carminative, depurative, detoxicant, diuretic, emmenagogue, relaxing, rubefacient, stimulant, stomachic, sudorific, tonic, vulnerary.

Ways to Use Juniper Essential Oil

Acne – juniper oil contains mild antiseptic properties which have a cleansing effect on acne skin. Mix 3 drops with 1 teaspoon of coconut, oil and massage into the face and neck. You can also add 1-2 drops to your moisturiser, and carry out your skincare routine normally. Repeat 3-4 times per week.

Arthritis – juniper oil has strong cleansing properties and therefore encourages the removal of uric acids, which is one of the main causes of arthritis. Mix 4 drops of juniper oil with 1 teaspoon of carrier oil, and massage into the affected area. You can also dilute 4 drops with 1 tablespoon of carrier oil, and add to a warm bath.

Cellulite – juniper oil's diuretic properties help to speed up the elimination of fluid retention, which eventually diminishes the appearance of cellulite. Mix 4 drops of the oil with 1 tablespoon of carrier oil, and massage into the affected area. Use firm movements with moderate pressure.

Dermatitis – juniper oil imparts soothing and antiseptic actions on the skin and helps to reduce inflammation and ease any pain associated with dermatitis. Due to its astringent properties it should be used in moderation when treating this skin disorder. Mix 3 drops with 1 teaspoon of coconut oil, and massage into the affected area. You can also dilute 4 drops of the oil with 1 tablespoon of carrier oil. and add to a warm bath.

Detox – with excellent cleansing properties, juniper oil is ideal to use during a detox. Mix 2 drops of the oil with 1 teaspoon of carrier oil, and massage into the feet. Repeat once per week for 4 weeks.

Fluid Retention – mix 4 drops of juniper oil with 1 tablespoon of carrier oil, and massage into the affected areas. Always massage towards the heart to encourage elimination.

Juniper is a powerful diuretic and should only be used when the fluid retention is not caused by lack of kidney function, as it can further irritate the kidneys.

Insomnia – juniper oil has excellent sedative and relaxing properties so diffusing 2 drops before bedtime will help you drift off into a peaceful sleep. You can also dilute 4 drops of the oil with 100ml of water, and spray onto your pillow before bedtime. Shake well before use.

Mental Fatigue – diffuse 2-3 drops of juniper oil as it helps to clear and stimulate the mind.

Oily Skin – mix 3 drops with 1 teaspoon of coconut oil, massage into the skin and leave for 10 minutes. Then gently wipe off with a warm face cloth. Use as a bi-weekly treatment.

Stress – place 1-2 drops on a tissue, and inhale throughout the day. Juniper oil's calming properties will promote peace and relaxation. You can also mix 2 drops with 1 teaspoon of carrier oil, and massage into the back of the neck and across the shoulders.

Lavender Oil

An all-rounder oil, lavender has a wealth of therapeutic actions that have a positive effect on both body and mind. Its excellent anti-inflammatory and antiseptic properties make it the go-to-oil for burns, insect bites, sunburn, bacterial and viral skin disorders, and athlete's foot. Lavender oil has a calming and balancing effect on both the parasympathetic and sympathetic nervous systems, therefore useful for treating insomnia, hyperactivity, stress, panic attacks, depression, restlessness, and anxiety.

Properties: analgesic, antidepressant, anti-inflammatory, antirheumatic, antiseptic, antispasmodic, antiviral, bactericide, calming, carminative, cholagogue, cicatrisant, cytophylactic, decongestant, deodorant, diuretic, emmenagogue, fungicide, hypotensive, nervine, relaxing, sedative, sudorific, vulnerary.

Ways to Use Lavender Essential Oil

Air Freshener – lavender oil has a beautiful, fresh aroma, and can therefore be used as an air freshener. Diffuse 4 drops, or place 2-3 drops on potpourri to keep it fresh.

Blemishes – apply 1 drop of lavender oil directly on a blemish or pimple to help destroy bacteria, reduce inflammation and redness, and prevent possible scarring.

Burns – in the event of a minor burn, immediately place 2-3 drops of lavender oil on the area. The lavender oil will relieve the pain and prevent a blister from forming. It may take 3-4 minutes for the stinging to subside but persevere with it as the results are fantastic.

Cystitis – to help relieve stinging, inflammation, and any pain associated with cystitis, mix 5 drops with 1 tablespoon of carrier oil, and add to a warm bath. Soak for 20 minutes.

Digestion – Mix 4 drops with 1 teaspoon of carrier oil, and massage into the abdomen. Lavender oil helps to stimulate digestion, acting as a tonic for the digestive tract as a whole.

Hyperactivity – whether you are suffering from a hyper or overactive mind or body, diffusing 4 drops of lavender oil can instil feelings of peace, calm, and relaxation. You can also dilute 5 drops with 1 teaspoon of carrier oil, and add to a warm bath.

Closet Freshener – place 2 drops of lavender oil on a cotton ball, and place in your closet to repel insects and moths. It also creates a pleasant, fresh scent.

Cold Sores – lavender oil contains powerful antiviral properties, which are effective in treating and healing cold sores. Place 1 drop of lavender oil directly onto a cold sore using a cotton swab. Repeat twice per day.

Dandruff – lavender oil is a good oil to use on dandruff as it helps to replenish lost moisture in the scalp, and it effectively clears dry, flaky skin. Mix 12 drops with 2 tablespoons of coconut oil, and massage onto a clean scalp. Leave for 40 minutes, and thoroughly rinse your hair.

Dry Skin Conditions – lavender oil is an effective treatment to use on dry skin conditions such as dermatitis and eczema. It helps to reduce inflamed skin, soothe irritation, and speed up the healing process. Mix 4 drops with 1 teaspoon of coconut oil, and massage into the area of concern. Repeat daily.

Earache – gently massage 1 drop of lavender oil behind each ear to help relieve the pain and discomfort of an earache. Never pour the oil directly into the eardrum.

Fabric Conditioner – place 4 drops of lavender oil in with your fabric conditioner to freshen clothes and create a beautiful, natural scent.

Fever – mix 4 drops with 1 teaspoon of carrier oil, and massage into the soles of the feet. You can also add 4 drops to a steam inhalation. Lavender oil helps to break the fever by reducing the temperature of the body. It also fights the infection.

Headaches – the analgesic action of lavender oil, together with its relaxing effect on the nervous system, makes it an effective treatment for headaches or migraines. Simply place 1 drop of lavender oil on each temple to ease any pain.

Healthy Hair – adding 4 drops of lavender oil to your conditioner helps to keep the hair healthy and strong.

Insect Bites & Bee Stings – put a drop of lavender directly on the sting or bite, and gently rub it in. Any itching or swelling will be reduced.

Insect Repellent – lavender oil successfully repels insects and bugs, and therefore makes for an effective natural insect repellent. Place 1 drop of lavender oil on each ankle, 1 drop behind each thigh, and 1 drop on each shoulder before going out in the evening. Alternatively, add 15 drops to a 200ml spray bottled filled with water, and spray over the upper and lower body regularly throughout the evening.

Insomnia – lavender oil has a calming effect on the nervous system, and is therefore an excellent choice for those suffering from insomnia. Place 2 drops on your pillow before bedtime, or diffuse 3 drops in your bedroom.

Linen Spray – add 15 drops of lavender oil to a 300ml spray bottle of filtered water, and spritz sheets, pillows, towels, and curtains to keep fabrics smelling fresh.

Menstrual Cramps – mix 4 drops with 1 teaspoon of carrier oil, and massage into the lower abdomen. Alternatively, add 3 drops to a hot compress, and drape across the abdomen. Lavender oil calms uterine spasms, and helps to ease the pain from cramping.

Motion Sickness – lavender oil helps to settle an upset tummy, and is effective at dispelling feelings of nausea. Place 2 drops on a tissue, and inhale regularly throughout your journey.

Muscular Aches & Pains – the anti-inflammatory and analgesic properties contained within lavender oil are beneficial to use on aching muscles. Dilute 7 drops of the oil with 1 tablespoon of carrier oil, and add to a warm bath. Alternatively, mix 5 drops with 1 tablespoon of carrier oil, and massage into affected muscles.

Rashes – lavender oil helps to reduced inflammation, ease the stinging of a rash, or alleviate itching. It also helps to protect pimples from becoming infected. Mix 5 drops with 1 tablespoon of coconut oil, and massage into the area of concern.

Scar Tissue – to reduce the appearance of scar tissue, mix 3 drops of lavender oil with 1 teaspoon of coconut oil, and massage into the area. This formula can also be used to minimize the formation of scar tissue on a recent cut or wound. Repeat twice per day.

Shingles – for large areas, mix 6-7 drops of lavender oil with 1 tablespoon of coconut oil, and massage into affected areas. For smaller areas, mix 3-4 drops with 1 teaspoon of coconut oil. Lavender oil possesses potent antiviral properties, helping to destroy the herpes virus, while also reducing inflammation and pain.

Sinusitis – lavender oil helps to clear congested nasal passageways, making breathing easier. Add 4 drops to a steam inhalation.

Stress & Tension – lavender oil is a fantastic stress reliever. It calms the body and mind, creating harmony and tranquillity. Place 2 drops on a tissue, and inhale regularly during stressful situations. You can also diffuse 4 drops of the oil, or add 15 drops to a 200ml spray bottle filled with water, and mist over the upper body when you feel the need.

Sunburn – lavender oil is very effective at calming the stinging and burning sensations of sunburn. It also helps to prevent blistering and any possible scarring. Mix 5 drops of the oil with 1 teaspoon of coconut oil, and gently massage into the area. You can also add 15 drops to a 200ml spray bottle filled with water, and spray over the area several times per day.

Swollen Feet – add 4 drops of lavender oil to a foot bath, and soak for 20 minutes. Lavender oil helps to ease swelling and stimulate blood circulation around the feet and ankles.

Toilet Roll Fragrance – place 2-3 drops of lavender oil on a new roll of toilet paper, and each time it is used, the fresh scent of lavender will be released into the bathroom.

Lemon Oil

A wonderful tonic for the skin, lemon oil helps to rejuvenate dull, tired skin, and is used to treat oily and acne skin. It has a refreshing and stimulating effect on the body and mind, allowing for mental clarity as well as an increase in energy levels. Lemon oil is a great tonic for the digestive system, helping to soothe indigestion, improve the absorption of nutrients around the body, and relieve flatulence and constipation. It is also an effective household cleaner and insect repellent.

Properties: antibacterial, antifungal, antimicrobial, antirheumatic, antiseptic, antispasmodic, astringent, carminative, cicatrisant, depurative, diaphoretic, digestive, diuretic, febrifuge, hypotensive, insecticidal, laxative, rubefacient, tonic, vermifuge.

Ways to Use Lemon Essential Oil

Age Spots – lemon oil helps to fade age spots when used regularly. Mix 1 drop of lemon oil with 1 drop of coconut oil, and massage onto the age spot 2-3 times per day.

Anxiety – if you are feeling anxious, place 2 drops of lemon oil on a tissue, and inhale regularly. You can also mix 5 drops of lemon oil with 1 teaspoon of carrier oil, and massage into the chest, shoulders, and back of the neck. Lemon oil can be very calming for those who suffer from anxiety.

Blisters – place a drop of lemon oil directly over a blister to ease swelling and redness.

Carpet Cleaner – place 8-10 drops of lemon oil into your carpet cleaner for a bright, stain-free rug.

Cellulite – mix 8 drops of lemon oil with 1 tablespoon of coconut oil, and firmly massage into problem areas. Lemon oil contains excellent diuretic properties, which increase the frequency of urination. This increase helps with the quicker removal of toxins, fats, and wastes from the body. Fatty deposits break up, and eventually the appearance of cellulite diminishes.

Corns & Calluses – lemon oil helps to heal, clear or prevent infection, and reduce any redness around corns or calluses. Mix 3 drops with 1 teaspoon of coconut oil, and massage into the affected area twice per day.

Coughs & Congestion – lemon oil's expectorant properties help to expel mucus build-up in the respiratory tract, ease coughing spasms, and relax breathing by calming the nervous system. Add 3 drops to a steam inhalation, or mix 4 drops with 1 teaspoon of carrier oil, and massage into the chest.

De-Greaser – lemon oil is an effective de-greaser. Whether on your hands or body, kitchen countertop or car, grease can be easily washed off by placing 2-3 drops of lemon oil in hot, soapy water.

Depression – lemon oil has a stimulating effect on the mind, helping to uplift the spirits and alleviate low moods. Diffuse 4 drops, or mix 4 drops with 1 teaspoon of carrier oil, and massage into the soles of the feet.

Dishwasher Detergent – add 1 drop of lemon oil to your dishwasher cleaner for spot free dishes. Alternatively, add 1 drop to your sink if you are hand washing dishes.

Fatigue – lemon oil invigorates the body and mind and helps to boost energy levels. Diffuse 4 drops, or mix 4 drops with 1 teaspoon of carrier oil, and massage into the soles of the feet.

Furniture Polish – lemon oil is an excellent homemade furniture polish made from 1 tablespoon of olive oil mixed with 4 drops of lemon oil. It creates a beautiful shine, moisturizes wood, and leaves behind a fresh, citrus smell.

Insect Repellent – diffuse 4 drops of lemon oil in the evening to repel mosquitoes and other bugs. Alternatively, place 1 drop on each ankle. Never use during the day due to the photosensitive nature of lemon oil.

Mental Clarity – diffuse 3 drop of lemon oil to refresh the brain and promote focus and concentration.

Metal Polisher – place 6-8 drops of lemon oil on a paper towel, and polish door handles, bathroom taps, and most metal surfaces. This will create shiny surfaces, and destroy any bacteria that may be present.

Sanitation – lemon oil can be used to sanitize the hands, whether after a bathroom visit, leaving a hospital, or after preparing food. Place 1 drop on the palm of the hands and rub the hands together.

Skincare – lemon oil is a fantastic treatment for dull, congested skin as it helps to clean and tighten pores, brighten the complexion, and remove dead skin cells. Mix 4 drops with 1 teaspoon of coconut oil, and massage into the face and neck. Alternatively, add 3 drops to a steam inhalation.

Surface Cleaner – add 12-15 drops of lemon oil into a 400ml spray bottle filled with water, and use to clean kitchen or bathroom surfaces. Lemon oil kills germs that linger in these areas and brightens surfaces.

Unpleasant Smells – a fantastic air freshener, lemon oil can be used to eliminate damp or mildew smells, or bad odors from food or animals. Diffuse 4 drops of the oil, or add 3 drops to a clean cloth, and polish smelly surfaces.

Varicose Veins – lemon oil stimulates the circulatory system, and therefore helps to improve blood circulation around the body. To help treat varicose veins, mix 4 drops of the oil with 1 teaspoon of coconut oil, and massage the limb in an upwards direction towards the heart. Never massage directly on the varicose veins, only on either side.

Lemongrass Oil

Due to the combination of its antibacterial and astringent properties, lemongrass oil is commonly used to treat oily, acne prone skin. It also revitalizes both body and mind, helping to ease aching muscles, soothe tired legs, relieve stress related conditions, and combat nervous exhaustion.

Properties: analgesic, antidepressant, antimicrobial, antiseptic, astringent, bactericidal, carminative, deodorant, febrifuge, fungicidal, galactagogue, insecticidal, nervine, sedative, stimulant, tonic, uplifting.

Ways to Use Lemongrass Essential Oil

Acne – mix 4 drops with 1 teaspoon of coconut oil, and massage into the face and neck. Alternatively, add 4 drops to a steam inhalation. The lemongrass oil will help draw out impurities from blemishes, prevent infection, and close dilated pores. Repeat 2-3 times per week.

Cellulite – lemongrass oil helps to increase urination, which helps to remove toxins and fat deposits in the body's tissues just under the surface of the skin, lessening the appearance of cellulite over time. Blend 6 drops of the oil with 1 tablespoon of coconut oil, and massage into the area of concern. Repeat daily.

Depression – dilute 7 drops in 1 tablespoon of carrier oil, and add to a warm bath. Alternatively, diffuse 5 drops of the oil, or blend 6 drops with 1 teaspoon of carrier oil, and massage into the feet. Lemongrass oil instils feelings of joy, hope, and optimism, helping to uplift spirits and fight depression.

Detox – lemongrass oil stimulates lymph drainage, helping with the efficient removal of toxins from the body. Dilute 7 drops of the oil in 1 tablespoon of carrier oil, and add to an Epsom salt bath. Soak for 20 minutes.

Emotional Support – lemongrass oil helps to revive, energize, and stimulate the emotions, creating balance when you feel 'out of sync'. Diffuse 5 drops in your home, or place 2 drops on a tissue, and inhale regularly throughout the day.

Energy Levels – mix 5 drops with 1 teaspoon of carrier oil, and massage into the feet to boost energy levels and build up a resistance to fatigue. Alternatively, diffuse 5 drops in your home to stimulate the nervous system.

Fever – lemongrass oil helps to reduce fever by fighting the infection that causes the actual fever. It also reduces high temperatures and induces sweating for faster elimination of toxins. Mix 7 drops with 2 tablespoons of carrier oil, and massage into the body. Alternatively, dilute 6 drops in 1 tablespoon of carrier oil, and add to an Epsom salt bath.

Flatulence – lemongrass oil provides relief from excess flatulence. Mix 4 drops with 1 teaspoon of carrier oil, and massage into the abdomen in a clockwise direction.

Fluid Retention – dilute 7 drops in 1 tablespoon of carrier oil, and add to an Epsom salt bath. Soak for 20 minutes. Lemongrass oil helps to remove excess fluid from the body and reduce any swelling. Repeat daily until swelling decreases.

Focus & Concentration – diffuse 5 drops of lemongrass oil to clear any sluggishness from the air. Lemongrass helps to clear the mind, and help with logical thinking and concentration.

Gums & Teeth – add 3 drops to a small amount of water, and use as a mouth wash. Do not swallow. Lemongrass oil helps by contracting the gums to promote strength and durability of the teeth.

Headaches – lemongrass oil provides relief from headaches. Mix 2 drops in ½ teaspoon of carrier oil, and massage into the temples, or diffuse 3 drops in the room.

Immune System – lemongrass oil acts as a tonic for the whole organism, treating and preventing infectious illnesses both internally and externally. Dilute 6 drops in 1 tablespoon of carrier oil, and add to a warm bath. Soak for 20 minutes. You can also create a massage oil for the body by blending 8 drops with 2 tablespoons of carrier oil.

Insect Repellent – lemongrass is a very effective insect repellent. Diffuse 6 drops and place the diffuser close by. or add 15 drops to a 300ml spray bottle of filtered water, and spray around your upper and lower body regularly throughout the evening.

Muscular Aches & Pains – mix 5 drops with 1 tablespoon of carrier oil, and massage into the affected area. Adding a dilution of 6 drops in 1 tablespoon of carrier oil to a warm bath will also help to soothe aching muscles and relieve pain.

Open Pores – lemongrass oil possesses potent astringent properties, making it a beneficial treatment to tighten pores and tone the skin. Mix 4 drops with 1 teaspoon of coconut oil, and massage into the face, paying particular attention to the forehead, nose, and chin. Repeat daily.

Parkinson's Disease – lemongrass oil acts as a tonic for the nervous system, strengthening and stimulating the nerves. It can ease shaking or trembling. Diffuse 5 drops, or mix 6 drops with 1 tablespoon of carrier oil, and massage on either side of the spine.

Poor Circulation – lemongrass oil improves the flow of blood through the body by dilating and strengthening blood vessels, and can therefore help with various venous conditions including varicose veins and chilblains. Mix 8 drops with 2 tablespoons of carrier oil, and massage into the body. Adding a dilution of 6 drops of the oil with 1 tablespoon of carrier oil to a bath will also help to improve circulation.

Rheumatism – lemongrass oil is a popular oil of choice for treating aches and pains, and any inflammation associated with rheumatism. Mix 8 drops with 2 tablespoons of carrier oil, and massage into the body. You can also add 5 drops to a hot compress and hold over the area of concern for 5-10 minutes.

Tired, Swollen Feet – dilute 5 drops of lemongrass oil in ½ tablespoon of carrier oil, and add to a foot bath. Alternatively, massage the formula directly into the feet. Lemongrass oil helps to soothe aching feet and reduce swollen, inflamed tissue.

Lime Oil

Lime oil has a stimulating effect on the mind, helping to uplift spirits, promote focus and concentration, clear mental exhaustion, and release negative thoughts. It helps to fight colds and flu due to its antiviral and antibacterial properties, and also relieves coughing, bronchitis, and asthma. Lime oil has a toning effect on oily skin, and helps to clear blemishes. It is often used as a household cleaner because of its strong disinfectant qualities.

Properties: antiseptic, antiviral, astringent, bactericide, disinfectant, febrifuge, hemostatic, insecticide, tonic.

Ways to Use Lime Essential Oil

Acne – lime oil contains antibacterial properties, which help to clear blemishes and prevent infections. It also possesses astringent properties, which reduce the appearance of enlarged pores. Add 3 drops to a steam inhalation, or mix 3 drops with 1 teaspoon of coconut oil, and massage into the face and neck.

Air Freshener – lime oil has a fresh, fruity odor and makes a great natural air freshener. Diffuse 5 drops in the home.

Bacterial Infections – lime oil is an excellent remedy for many bacterial infections including impetigo, boils, and carbuncles. It contains antibacterial properties, which help to destroy the infection and heal the skin. Mix 2 drops with ½ teaspoon of coconut oil, and dab onto the affected area twice per day. You can also add 2 drops to a cold compress, and hold over the infection for 5 minutes.

Bleeding – lime oil helps to contract blood vessels and encourage the formation of blood clots on an open wound. Add 2 drops to a cold compress, and drape over the cut or wound.

Cellulite – lime oil stimulates the circulation of wastes and toxins through the lymphatic system at a quicker rate, which means they do not accumulate in the tissues of the body and create cellulite. Mix 5 drops with 1 tablespoon of coconut oil, and firmly massage into the areas of concern.

Chicken Pox – lime oil's powerful antiviral properties make it a beneficial oil to use when suffering from chicken pox. It helps to fight the infection and keep the pimples clean. Mix 5 drops with 1 tablespoon of carrier oil, and dab over the virus twice per day.

Cleansing Agent – the disinfectant, antibacterial, and antiseptic properties found in lime oil make it an extremely effective natural household cleaner. Add 20 drops to a 500ml spray bottle filled with filtered water, and use to clean surfaces in the kitchen and bathroom. Shake well before use.

Colds & Flu – lime oil can help to fight colds and flu by reducing the infection. Diffuse 5 drops, or add 3 drops to a steam inhalation.

Cold Sores – mix 2 drops of lime oil with ½ teaspoon of coconut oil, and dab part of the blend directly onto the cold sore using a cotton bud. Repeat 2-3 times per day. This works best when you catch the cold sore at the beginning tingling stage. Lime oil is effective at fighting viral infections.

Depression – mix 4 drops with 1 teaspoon of carrier oil, and massage into the feet. You can also diffuse 5 drops in your home to alleviate low moods and create hope and optimism.

Energy Levels – diffusing 5 drops of lime oil helps to boost energy levels and uplift the spirits. You can also place 2 drops on a tissue, and inhale regularly throughout the day.

Fever – lime oil's antiviral and antibacterial properties support the immune system in fighting the infection that causes fever. Add 3 drops to a steam inhalation, or add 3 drops to a cold compress and drape across the forehead or chest.

Gum Ulcer – use as a mouth wash to help cure gum ulcers. Add 2 drops to a small mouthful of water, and swirl around the mouth for 60 seconds. Do not swallow.

Hair Loss – dilute 6 drops in 1 tablespoon of olive or coconut oil, and massage into the scalp. Leave for 30 minutes and wash hair as normal. Lime oil has a tightening and toning effect on the scalp, which can reduce hair loss.

Mental Clarity – lime oil helps the mind to concentrate and focus, easing a fatigued, tired mind. Diffuse 5 drops, or place 2 drops on a tissue, and inhale regularly.

Mumps or Measles – lime oil contains excellent antiviral and antiseptic properties that help to fight the infection that caused mumps or measles, and prevent them from spreading. Mix 5 drops with 1 tablespoon of coconut oil, and dab the blend over the skin lesions. Repeat twice per day 2-3 times per week followed by a week off.

Oily Skin – lime oil is useful for treating oily skin as it helps to balance the production of sebum in the skin and also helps to cleanse and tighten pores. Mix 3 drops with 1 teaspoon of coconut oil, and massage into the face and neck.

Shingles – mix 5 drops with 1 tablespoon of coconut oil, and massage over the rash. Lime oil helps to clear the rash and also contains antiseptic properties, which will keep it clean and prevent it from spreading.

Skin Rash – lime oil is very effective at curing skin rashes resulting from allergies or internal infection due to its antiviral, antibacterial, and disinfectant properties. Mix 5 drops with 1 tablespoon of coconut oil, and massage over the rash. Increase or decrease the dosage depending on how many parts of the body are affected.

Throat Infections – lime oil's antimicrobial properties help to clear throat infections when taken internally. Add 2 drops to a small amount of water and gargle for 30 seconds. Repeat twice per day. Do not swallow.

Mandarin Oil

Mandarin oil is a refreshing and soothing oil. It helps to treat stretch marks, cellulite, and edema. It has powerful antispasmodic properties making it a great oil to use to relieve muscle cramps and stiffness. It also helps to calm and alleviate acne prone skin.

Properties: antispasmodic, antiviral, carminative, cholagogue, depurative, digestive, diuretic, relaxing, sedative, uplifting.

Ways to Use Mandarin Essential Oil

Coughs – mandarin oil helps to reduce spasms in the respiratory tract, which can cause persistent coughing. Add 3 drops to a steam inhalation, and breathe deeply for 3 minutes. You can also mix 4 drops with 1 teaspoon of carrier oil, and massage into the upper chest area.

Detox – mandarin oil helps to purify the blood, which helps to get rid of unwanted toxins from the body. Mix 4 drops with 1 teaspoon of carrier oil, and massage into the soles of the feet. You can also create a detox bath by diluting 6 drops in 1 tablespoon of carrier oil and, add to a warm Epsom salt bath.

Digestion – mandarin oil has a stimulating effect on the stomach, encouraging the secretion of digestive juices and bile to promote the efficient digestion of food. Mix 4 drops with 1 teaspoon of carrier oil, and massage into the abdomen in a clockwise direction.

Immune System - mix 4 drops with 1 teaspoon of carrier oil, and massage into the feet. Mandarin oil acts as a tonic for the body as a whole, helping to strengthen the immune system and protect it from illnesses such as colds and flu.

Liver Function – mix 4 drops with 1 teaspoon of carrier oil, and massage into the feet. Mandarin oil acts as a tonic for the liver, helping to strengthen and protect it from infections.

Oily Skin – mandarin oil acts as an astringent for oily skin, helping to close pores and tighten the skin. Mix 3 drops with 2 teaspoon of coconut oil, and massage into the face, paying particular attention to the t-zone area.

Scar Tissue – mandarin oil promotes the growth of new skin cells, thereby helping to fade the appearance of scars over time. Mix 3 drops of the oil with ½ teaspoon of coconut oil, and gently massage over scar tissue twice per day.

Stress & Anxiety – mandarin oil has a calming effect on the nervous system, helping to relax and overcome feelings of stress, tension, or anxiety. Diffuse 5 drops in your home, or place 2 drops on a tissue, and inhale regularly throughout the day during times of need.

Stretch Marks – the regular use of mandarin oil helps to both prevent and diminish the appearance of stretch marks. Mix 3 drops with 1 teaspoon of coconut oil, and massage into the area of concern. Repeat daily.

Vomiting – mix 4 drops with 1 teaspoon of carrier oil, and massage into the abdomen in a clockwise direction. Mandarin oil eases spasms in the intestines which cause vomiting.

Manuka Oil

The analgesic, antibacterial, antifungal, and anti-inflammatory properties contained within manuka oil make it a valuable oil when treating various skin disorders such as athlete's foot, rashes, acne, ulcers, cuts and abrasions, insect bites and stings, ringworm, psoriasis, dermatitis, and impetigo. Its analgesic effect is recommended for the relief of arthritis and rheumatism. Wound healing is significantly increased when using manuka oil.

Properties: analgesic, antibacterial, antifungal, anti-inflammatory, deodorant, expectorant, insecticide, sedative.

Ways to Use Manuka Essential Oil

Allergies – manuka oil is anti-allergenic, therefore easing allergic reactions, and in some cases preventing them from occurring altogether. Mix 4 drops with 1 teaspoon of carrier oil, and massage into the soles of the feet, or diffuse 4 drops in your home.

Arthritis & Rheumatism – manuka oil is an excellent treatment for joint pain as it helps to reduce inflammation around the joint, and also contains effective pain relieving properties. Mix 3 drops with 1 teaspoon of carrier oil, and massage into areas of concern. Alternatively, add 3 drops to a hot compress, and wrap around the affected area for 20 minutes.

Athlete's Foot – the antifungal capabilities of manuka oil are very powerful, and are therefore effective at treating athlete's foot. Mix 4 drops with 1 teaspoon of coconut oil, and massage into the foot and toes. Alternatively, add 4 drops to a foot bath, and soak for 30 minutes.

Bacterial Infections – manuka oil helps to prevent bacterial infections from taking place in the body due to its potent antibacterial properties. Diffuse 4 drops, or dilute 6 drops in 1 tablespoon of carrier oil, and add to a warm bath.

Boils & Folliculitis – manuka oil has excellent healing capabilities, along with a strong antiseptic action that makes it an excellent treatment for bacterial infections such as boils and folliculitis. Mix 2 drops with ½ teaspoon of coconut oil, and dab on the area 2-3 times per day.

Bronchitis – the decongestant action of manuka oil is beneficial for the treatment of bronchitis as it helps to relieve breathing by clearing air passageways of mucus build up.

Mix 4 drops with 1 teaspoon of carrier oil, and massage into the chest, or add 3 drops to a steam inhalation.

Colds & Flu – manuka oil not only helps to destroy the cold or flu virus, but it also acts as an expectorant to keep the respiratory tract free from phlegm and mucus. Add 4 drops to a steam inhalation, or mix 4 drops with 1 teaspoon of carrier oil, and massage into the chest.

Cold Sores – the strong antiviral action of manuka oil makes it an effective treatment for the cold sore virus. Mix 2 drops with ½ teaspoon of coconut oil, and dab onto the sore twice per day using a clean cotton swab each time.

Coughing – manuka oil is effective at clearing a persistent cough by helping to expel mucus build up in the air passageways. Mix 4 drops with 1 teaspoon of carrier oil, and massage into the chest.

Cuts & Wounds – manuka oil possesses powerful antiseptic properties which help to keep cuts and wounds clean and infection free. It is also an effective wound healer. Add 2 drops to a cold compress, and drape over the affected area. Alternatively, mix 2 drops with ½ teaspoon of coconut oil, and dab over the cut or wound.

Dandruff – Mix 5 drops with 1 tablespoon of coconut oil, and massage onto the scalp. Leave for 30 minutes and rinse off. Manuka oil helps to replenish lost moisture in the scalp and rid the area of dry, flaky skin.

Impetigo – mix 2 drops with ½ teaspoon of coconut oil, and dab over the area twice per day using a clean cotton swab. The antibacterial and antimicrobial properties contained within manuka oil help to clear this skin infection and prevent it from spreading.

Insect Bites & Stings – applying a small drop of manuka oil to an insect bite or sting will quickly reduce any pain and swelling around the area.

Insect Repellent – diffuse 4 drops of manuka oil, or add 20 drops to a 300ml spray bottle of filtered water, and spray around the ankles, knees, elbows, and shoulders. Manuka oil is an effective insecticide effectively working to keep insects at bay.

Muscular Aches & Pains – mix 5 drops with 1 tablespoon of carrier oil, and massage into the area of concern. Alternatively, dilute 6 drops in 1 tablespoon of carrier oil, and add to a warm bath. Manuka oil helps to reduce inflammation in the muscle and also eases aches and pain.

Rashes – manuka oil helps to calm rashes by alleviating inflammation and easing any pain experienced with this skin disorder. It also helps to protect lesions from becoming infected. Add 20 drops to a 300ml spray bottle of filtered water, and spray over the rash twice per day.

Ringworm – manuka oil has the ability to destroy the fungal infection that causes ringworm. It helps to reduce any inflammation and also speeds up the healing of the skin. Mix 4 drops with 1 teaspoon of coconut oil, and massage over the area of concern. Alternatively, add 3 drops to a cold compress, and drape across the affected area for 20 minutes.

Scar Tissue – manuka oil possesses excellent cell regeneration properties which promote the growth of new skin cells, reducing the appearance of scars over time. Mix 2 drops with 1 teaspoon of coconut oil, and massage over the scar twice per day.

Shingles – manuka oil is effective at eliminating viral infections, helping to not only destroy the virus, but reduce inflammation and ease any pain. Mix 5 drops with 1 tablespoon of coconut oil, and very gently dab onto breakout areas. Repeat twice per day.

Stress – manuka oil has a relaxing effect on the body and can help reduce stress or anxiety in times of need. Diffuse 4 drops, or place 2 drops on a tissue, and inhale regularly.

Marjoram Oil

With excellent warming and soothing properties, marjoram oil helps to ease joint pain and muscle spasms, relieves menstrual cramps, lowers high blood pressure, and eases indigestion. It also has a calming effect on emotions, easing stress and soothing the mind.

Properties: analgesic, anaphrodisiac, antiseptic, antispasmodic, antiviral, bactericidal, carminative, diaphoretic, digestive, diuretic, emmenagogue, expectorant, fungicidal, hypotensive, laxative, nervine, relaxing sedative, stomachic, vasodilator, vulnerary, warming.

Ways to Use Marjoram Essential Oil

Arthritis – marjoram oil soothes joint inflammations and is extremely effective at lessening any pain associated with arthritis. Mix 5 drops with 1 tablespoon of carrier oil, and massage into the affected limb, paying particular attention to the joints.

Bereavement – marjoram oil is beneficial for treating individuals in times of grief. It helps to soothe and calm the senses, warm the emotions, and instil feelings of hope. Diffuse 5 drops in times of need.

Brain Health – marjoram oil helps strengthen the brain, therefore reducing the chance of forgetfulness with advancing age. Diffuse 5 drops of the oil, or mix 4 drops with 1 teaspoon of carrier oil, and massage on either side of the spine and across the shoulders.

Coughing – diffuse 5 drops of marjoram oil, or mix 4 drops with 1 teaspoon of carrier oil, and massage into the chest area. Alternatively, add 3 drops to a steam inhalation, and inhale deeply for 2-3 minutes. Marjoram oil provides relief from respiratory spasms and helps to clear mucus and phlegm from the respiratory tract.

Flatulence – marjoram oil relaxes the muscles of the abdominals, ensuring there is no build up of gas in this area. Mix 5 drops of the oil with 1 tablespoon of carrier oil, and massage into the abdomen in a clockwise direction.

High Blood Pressure – marjoram oil dilates blood vessels, regulating the flow of blood. Mix 5 drops with 1 tablespoon of carrier oil. Massage over the heart center and into both feet.

Indigestion – mix 5 drops with 1 tablespoon of carrier oil, and massage into the chest and stomach area. Marjoram oil helps to regulate the secretion of gastric juices, bile, and stomach acids, helping to ensure the proper function of the digestive system.

Insomnia – place 2 drops on your pillow just before bedtime. or diffuse 4 drops in your bedroom. You can also add a dilution of 5 drops to 1 tablespoon of carrier oil to a warm bath before bedtime. Marjoram oil sedates the nervous system, thereby producing a calm and relaxed mind and body.

Irregular Periods – marjoram oil's emmenagogue properties means that it can stimulate blood flow in the uterine area and regulate the flow of menstruation. Mix 5 drops of the oil with 1 tablespoon of carrier oil, and massage into the abdomen in a clockwise direction. Alternatively, add 5 drops to a hot compress, and drape across the abdomen for 10 to 15 minutes.

Menstrual Cramps – marjoram oil helps to ease menstrual cramps as it acts as a muscle relaxant and has effective pain relieving properties. Mix 4 drops with 1 tablespoon of carrier oil, and massage into the lower abdomen and lower back.

Migraines – marjoram oil helps to reduce the pain of a migraine, but only use in small quantities so it does not overpower the senses. Diffuse 2 drops in your home, or mix 2 drops with 1 teaspoon of carrier oil, and massage into the temples and back of the neck.

Muscular Aches & Pains – mix 5 drops of marjoram oil with 1 tablespoon of carrier oil, and massage into the affected area. You can also dilute 5 drops in 1 tablespoon of carrier oil, and add to a warm bath. Marjoram oil eases tight, painful muscles due to its analgesic and warming properties.

Muscular Cramps – marjoram oil has excellent antispasmodic properties, and therefore provides relief from muscle cramps or muscle strain. Mix 6 drops of the oil with 1 tablespoon of carrier oil, and massage into the affected area. Alternatively, dilute 6 drops in 1 tablespoon of carrier oil, and add to a bath of warm water. If you suffer from leg cramps at night, repeat this treatment each night before bedtime.

Poor Circulation – marjoram oil dilates blood vessels, helping to improve sluggish circulation around the body. Dilute 6 drops in 1 tablespoon of carrier oil, and add to a warm bath. Immediately after the bath, stand under a cool shower for 20 seconds to further stimulate blood circulation.

Sex Drive – because marjoram oil lessens our physical and emotional response to situations, it has been known to suppress a sex drive or lessen any sexual urges. Diffuse 5 drops of the oil, or place 2 drops on a tissue, and inhale when you feel the need.

Sinusitis – marjoram oil eases congested nasal passageways, relieving the symptoms of sinusitis. Mix 4 drops of the oil with 1 teaspoon of carrier oil, and massage on either side of the nose and behind both ears. You can also diffuse 4 drops in your home to clear the air.

Stress & Tension – diffuse 6 drops of marjoram oil, or dilute 6 drops with 1 tablespoon of carrier oil, and add to a warm bath. Marjoram oil has a warming action on both the body and mind, helping to relieve anxiety and stress.

Toothache – mix 3 drops of marjoram oil with ½ teaspoon of carrier oil, and massage the blend into the area of the jaw where you feel the pain. It can reduce any inflammation associated with a toothache, and also ease the pain.

Vomiting – mix 5 drops with 1 tablespoon of carrier oil, and massage into the abdomen in a clockwise direction. Marjoram oil helps to lessen intestinal cramps, which can cause vomiting.

Wounds & Cuts – marjoram oil's powerful antiseptic properties ensure that wounds are protected against infection and are healed at a faster rate. Mix 2 drops of the oil with 1 teaspoon of coconut oil, and gently massage over the affected area. Repeat 2-3 times per day.

Melissa oil

Also known as lemon balm, this oil has a calming and uplifting effect on the body. It has fantastic antiviral and antibacterial properties making it an effective treatment for herpes, fungal infections, ulcers, and urinary tract infections. It also contains potent antidepressant properties and as a result, helps to lift moods and emotionally restore balance.

Properties: antidepressant, antispasmodic, antiviral, bactericidal, carminative, diaphoretic, emmenagogue, febrifuge, hypotensive, nervine, sedative, stomachic, sudorific, tonic.

Ways to Use Melissa Essential Oil

Allergies – whether of the skin or respiratory system, allergies can be treated effectively using Melissa oil. Mix 3 drops with 1 teaspoon of carrier oil, and massage into the feet.

Bacterial Infection – Melissa oil has excellent bactericidal properties which help to fight the infection and prevent it from spreading. Mix 2 drops with 1 teaspoon of coconut oil, and gently apply over the affected area twice per day.

Bronchitis – Melissa oil helps to ease coughing attacks often experienced during bronchitis. Add 2 drops to a steam inhalation, or mix 2 drops with 1 teaspoon of carrier oil and, massage into the chest area.

Colds &Flu – Melissa oil helps to induce sweating, which cools the body down during illness, and also helps to relieve congestion and calm coughing. Mix 3 drops with 1 teaspoon of carrier oil, and massage into the chest area, or add 2 drops to a steam inhalation.

Cold Sores – mix 1 drop of Melissa oil with 1 drop of coconut oil, and dab onto the cold sore 2-3 times per day. Melissa oil has the ability to fight viral infections and can prevent the cold sore from developing if used as soon you feel the tingle.

Depression – Melissa oil helps to lift the spirits, instilling feelings of hope and optimism. Diffuse 3 drops to dispel negative energy, or mix 2 drops with 1 teaspoon of carrier oil, and massage into the feet.

Digestion – Melissa oil helps to promote healthy digestion by regulating the secretion of digestive juices and bile in the stomach. Mix 3 drops with 1 teaspoon of carrier oil, and massage into the abdomen in a clockwise direction.

Fever – Melissa oil promotes perspiration, which cools the body temperature down during fever. It also helps to fight the infection that caused the fever to begin with. Mix 3 drops with 1 teaspoon of carrier oil, and massage into the feet. You can also add 8 drops to a spray mist, and spray over the face and upper body.

Flatulence – mix 3 drops with 1 teaspoon of carrier oil, and massage into the abdomen in a clockwise direction. Melissa oil helps to expel gases that build up in the intestines, relieving cramping and/or bloating.

Heart Palpitations – Melissa oil helps to calm an over rapid heartbeat, easing palpitations. Mix 2 drops with 1 teaspoon of carrier oil, and massage over the heart area, or diffuse 3 drops.

High Blood Pressure – Melissa oil acts as a tonic for the heart, helping to lower high blood pressure and therefore protect against heart attack. Mix 3 drops with 1 teaspoon of carrier oil, and massage over the heart area.

Insect Bites & Stings – Melissa oil helps to reduce inflamed skin around insect bites or sting, and ease stinging and itching. Mix 2 drops with 1 teaspoon of coconut oil, and dab onto the affected area 2-3 times per day.

Insomnia – place 1 drop on your pillow before bedtime, or diffuse 2 drops 10 minutes before you sleep. Melissa oil acts as a natural tranquilizer for both the body and mind, and helps to promote a good night's sleep.

Irregular Menstruation – mix 3 drops of Melissa oil with 1 teaspoon of carrier oil, and massage into the lower abdomen in a clockwise direction. Melissa oil has a mild emmenagogue action, thus normalizing irregular periods.

Menstrual Cramps – Melissa oil helps to reduce spasms in the uterine wall, reducing cramps. Mix 3 drops with 1 teaspoon of carrier oil, and massage into the abdomen in a clockwise direction.

Migraines & Headaches – Melissa oil calms the nerves in our brain, helping to ease the pain caused by headaches or migraines. Mix 1 drops with ½ teaspoon of carrier oil, and massage into the temples and back of the neck.

Nausea & Vomiting – Melissa oil's antispasmodic proprieties calm spasms in the stomach which can cause vomiting. Mix 2 drops of the oil with 1 teaspoon of carrier oil, and massage into the abdomen in a clockwise direction. You can also place 1 drop on a tissue, and inhale regularly when needed.

Nervous Tension & Anxiety – Melissa oil has a calming and soothing effect on the nervous system, helping to reduce nervous tension and ease an over-anxious mind. Add 10 drops to a spray mist, and spray over the upper body when you feel the need. You can also diffuse 3 drops, or place 1–2 drops on a tissue, and inhale regularly.

Shingles – Melissa oil possesses potent antiviral properties which help to clear the shingles virus. Mix 3 drops with 1 teaspoon of coconut oil, and apply directly over the lesions twice per day.

Shock – Melissa oil helps to calm the body in times of shock by reducing over-rapid breathing and heartbeat. Place 1-2 drops of the oil on a tissue, and inhale regularly, or diffuse 3 drops in your home.

Myrrh Oil

Containing powerful healing properties, myrrh oil soothes chapped or cracked skin, eases the symptoms of eczema or psoriasis, alleviates rashes, and treats stretch marks. It is also good for healing fungal infections such as ringworm, athlete's foot, and thrush. It has a warm, woody aroma, which leaves the body feeling uplifted.

Properties: anticatarrhal, anti-inflammatory, antimicrobial, antispasmodic, antiseptic, astringent, carminative, cicatrisant, digestive, emmenagogue, expectorant, fungicidal, sedative, stomachic, tonic, uterine, vulnerary.

Ways to Use Myrrh Essential Oil

Aging Skin – myrrh oil helps to reduce fine lines and wrinkles, and rejuvenates mature skin. Mix 5 drops with 1 teaspoon of coconut oil, and massage into the face and neck. Repeat 3 times per week with 1 week on and 1 week off.

Athlete's Foot – mix 4 drops with 1 teaspoon of coconut oil, and massage into clean feet, making sure you massage in between the toes. Myrrh oil not only helps to fight the fungus infection but also calms any itching or inflammation and soothes chapped, flaky skin.

Bronchitis – myrrh oil helps to dry up excess mucus and reduce inflammation, making it an effective treatment for bronchitis. Mix 4 drops of the oil with 1 teaspoon of carrier oil, and massage into the chest and throat area. Alternatively, add 4 drops to a steam inhalation, or simply diffuse 5 drops in your room.

Colds & Flu – myrrh oil helps to relieve congestion and fight the viral infection that causes a cold or flu. Diffuse 5 drops of the oil, or add 4 drops to a steam inhalation. You can also mix 5 drops with 1 teaspoon of carrier oil, and massage into the chest area.

Coughing – myrrh oil is highly valued as a healer of respiratory disorders. Its anticatarrhal and expectorant properties help to expel mucus from the lungs and reduce an inflamed respiratory tract. Add 4 drops to a steam inhalation. Alternatively, diffuse 5 drops in your home, or create a chest salve by mixing 4 drops with 1 teaspoon of carrier oil, and massage into the chest area.

Cracked Heels – myrrh oil's antibacterial, anti-inflammatory, antiseptic, and antifungal qualities mean cracked heels can be treated effectively and healed at a faster rate. Mix 3 drops with 1 teaspoon of coconut oil, and massage into the cracked heels. Repeat daily for 1 week on, 1 week off.

Detox – myrrh oil facilitates the removal of toxins and wastes from the body, keeping the immune system healthy and strong. Dilute 6 drops with 1 tablespoon of carrier oil, and add to an Epsom salt bath. You can also mix 4 drops with 1 teaspoon of carrier oil, and massage into the feet.

Digestion – myrrh oil promotes efficient digestion by stimulating the secretion of gastric juices and bile in the stomach. Mix 5 drops with 1 tablespoon of carrier oil, and massage into the abdomen in a clockwise direction.

Eczema – mix 4 drops of myrrh oil with 1 teaspoon of coconut oil, and massage into the affected area. For larger areas, mix 6 drops with 1 tablespoon. Myrrh oil helps to heal eczema at a faster rate by relieving itching, soothing chapped skin, and reducing inflammation. Repeat 2-3 times per week for 1 week on and 1 week off.

Flatulence – myrrh oil acts as a tonic for the digestive system, helping to relieve any gas build-up in the intestines. Mix 5 drops with 1 tablespoon of carrier oil, and massage into the abdomen in a clockwise direction.

Gingivitis – myrrh oil has potent gum healing capabilities, particularly healing for gingivitis. Add 3 drops to a small amount of water, and use as a mouth rinse. Do not swallow.

Lack of Motivation – diffuse 5 drops of myrrh oil in your home, or mix 4 drops with 1 teaspoon of carrier oil, and massage into the chest and across the shoulders. Myrrh oil helps to revive the nervous system, creating an alert, stimulated mind.

Menstrual Cramps – myrrh oil helps to ease the pain of menstrual cramps and regulates the menstrual cycle. Mix 5 drops with 1 tablespoon of carrier oil, and massage into the abdomen and lower back.

Mouth Ulcers – add 3 drops of myrrh oil to a small amount of water and use as a mouth rinse. Do not swallow. Also add 1 drop of the oil to a small amount of aloe vera gel and apply over the ulcer. Leave on for 5 minutes and rinse the mouth. Do not swallow.

PMS – diffuse 5 drops of myrrh oil, or blend 4 drops with 1 teaspoon of carrier oil, and massage into the soles of the feet. Myrrh oil helps to regulate any hormonal imbalance and instils feelings of peace and harmony.

Rashes – mix 7 drops of myrrh oil with 2 tablespoons of coconut oil, and massage into the body. Myrrh oil eases itching and reduces inflammation. It will also help to prevent any pimples from becoming infected.

Ringworm – the fungicidal properties contained within myrrh oil help to fight the fungus infection that cause ringworm. Mix 6 drops with 2 tablespoons of carrier oil, and massage into the body. You can also dilute 4 drops in 1 tablespoon of carrier oil, and add to a warm bath.

Scar Tissue – myrrh oil helps to fade scar tissue over time due to its ability to promote healthy new cells. Mix 4 drops with 1 teaspoon of coconut oil, and gently massage into scar tissue. Repeat daily for 1 week on, 1 week off.

Stretch Marks – myrrh oil's skin regenerating properties makes it a beneficial treatment for the prevention of stretch marks. Regular use will also reduce the appearance of stretch marks. Mix 4 drops with 1 teaspoon of coconut oil, and massage into the affected area. Use every day for 1 week and then change to another suitable oil such as neroli or lavender. Use myrrh oil for 2 weeks out of the month.

Vaginal Thrush – add 2 drops onto a cold compress, and hold over the affected area for 3 minutes. Alternatively, you can mix 3 drops of the oil with 1 teaspoon of coconut oil, and massage into the soles of the feet and heels. Myrrh oil helps to fight the fungus infection that causes thrush.

Myrtle Oil

The astringent properties contained within myrtle oil make it a beneficial treatment for oily skin, acne, hemorrhoids, weak gums, and enlarged pores. It has an excellent anticatarrhal action on the body and is therefore useful for treating bronchitis, coughing, colds & flu, and nasal congestion. Urinary tract infections, cystitis, and leucorrhea can also be treated effectively with this oil.

Properties: anticatarrhal, antiseptic, astringent, bactericidal, expectorant, sedative, tonic.

Ways to Use Myrtle Essential Oil

Acne – the astringent and antiseptic properties found in myrtle oil help to treat acne by tightening enlarged pores and clearing up blemishes. Mix 3 drops with 1 teaspoon of coconut oil, and massage into the face and neck twice per day.

Aphrodisiac – diffusing 4 drops of myrtle oil can help increase sexual desire and help alleviate impotency and frigidity.

Bladder Infections – dilute 4 drops in 1 tablespoon of carrier oil, and add to a sitz bath. Myrtle oil contains antiseptic properties, which help to treat bladder infections.

Bronchitis – myrtle oil is very effective at relieving bronchitis as it helps to clear mucus or catarrh build-up from the respiratory tract, making breathing easier. Add 3 drops to a steam inhalation, or mix 4 drops with 1 teaspoon of carrier oil, and massage into the chest area.

Coughing – mix 4 drops with 1 teaspoon of carrier oil, and massage into the chest, or diffuse 4 drops. Myrtle oil provides good relief from coughing as it breaks up phlegm and mucus in the lungs.

Cuts & Wounds – myrtle oil is a good oil to use on cuts and wounds to help keep them clean and prevent any infection from taking place. Add 2 drops to a cold compress, and hold over the area for 5 minutes. Repeat twice per day.

Hemorrhoids – the astringent properties contained within myrtle oil encourage the contraction of blood vessels and can therefore help to treat hemorrhoids effectively. Dilute 5 drops in 1 tablespoon of carrier oil, and add to a warm bath. Soak for 20 minutes.

Oily Skin – myrtle oil contains astringent properties, which have a beneficial effect on oily skin, helping to tighten pores and tone the skin. Mix 3 drops with 1 teaspoon of coconut oil, and massage into the face and neck, or add 3 drops to a steam inhalation.

Sinusitis – myrtle oil helps to clear congestion in the nasal passageways, providing relief from blocked sinuses. Add 3 drops to a steam inhalation, or diffuse 4 drops.

Stress – myrtle oil is sedative in nature and can therefore have a calming effect on the body and mind. Diffuse 4 drops in the home.

Niaouli Oil

Niaouli oil has effective skin healing capabilities, and is therefore useful when treating acne, blemishes, ulcers, boils, minor burns, abrasions, insect bites, and cuts. It acts as a respiratory tonic, helping to relieve asthma, bronchitis, sinusitis, coughs, colds, flu, sore throats, and chest infections. The analgesic properties found in niaouli oil help to relieve the pain of neuralgia, arthritis, and rheumatism.

Properties: analgesic, antirheumatic, antiseptic, bactericide, cicatrisant, decongestant, febrifuge, insecticide, stimulant, vermifuge, vulnerary.

Ways to Use Niaouli Essential Oil

Blocked Nose – niaouli oil is an expectorant and decongestant, therefore helping to clear congestion and relieve blocked nasal passageways. Add 3 drops to a steam inhalation, or mix 4 drops with 1 teaspoon of carrier oil, and massage into the upper chest and each side of the nose.

Chest Infection – mix 4 drops with 1 teaspoon of carrier oil, and massage into the chest area. Alternatively, add 3 drops to a steam inhalation, and repeat twice per day. Niaouli oil helps to expel mucus and phlegm that has accumulated in the respiratory tract.

Concentration – diffuse 5 drops of niaouli oil, or mix 3 drops with 1 teaspoon of carrier oil, and massage into the upper chest. Niaouli oil helps to clear the mind and encourage focus and mental clarity.

Fatigue – niaouli oil is a powerful stimulant helping to awaken the senses and boost energy levels. Place 2 drops on a tissue, and inhale regularly, or diffuse 5 drops in the home to clear sluggish air.

Fever – niaouli oil helps to reduce the temperature of the body and fight the infection that caused the fever to begin with. Diffuse 5 drops of the oil, or add 10 drops to 300ml of water in a spray bottle. Spray several times per day. Keep the bottle in a cool place and shake well before use.

Immunity – niaouli oil encourages the absorption of nutrients in the body, therefore helping to keep the immune system strong and supported. Mix 4 drops with 1 teaspoon of carrier oil, and massage into the feet.

Impetigo – mix 1 drop of niaouli oil with 1 drop of coconut oil, and apply directly over the infection using a cotton bud. Niaouli oil helps to clean the infection and prevent it spreading to other areas of the face and body.

Insect Repellent – diffuse 5 drops of the oil to help keep pesky insects at bay.

Jet Lag – niaouli oil possesses potent stimulating properties and can be used effectively to treat fatigue and lack of energy experienced during jet lag. Place 2 drops on a tissue, and inhale regularly, or add 10 drops to 300ml of water in a spray bottle, and spray around the upper body throughout the day. Shake well before use.

Mature Skin – niaouli oil speeds up the regeneration of skin cells which help fight signs of aging and refresh an otherwise dull complexion. Mix 4 drops with 1 teaspoon of coconut oil, and massage into the face and neck.

Muscular Pain – niaouli oil's powerful pain relieving capabilities make it an effective treatment for muscle aches and pains, including muscle strain or post exercise pain. Mix 5 drops with 1 tablespoon of carrier oil, and massage into the muscle. You can also dilute 6 drops in 1 tablespoon of carrier oil, and add to a warm bath.

Nerve Pain – mix 4 drops with 1 teaspoon of carrier oil, and gently massage over the area of concern. Niaouli oil is a powerful analgesic and helps to relieve pain by anaesthetizing nerves. Repeat daily.

Rheumatism – niaouli oil soothes and warms painful joints and is an effective pain reliever. Mix 4 drops with 1 teaspoon of carrier oil, and massage into the joints. Alternatively, add 4 drops to a hot compress and wrap around the area of pain.

Toothaches – mix 3 drops with 1 teaspoon of coconut oil, and massage along the jaw line and behind the ear. Niaouli oil helps to relieve the pain of a toothache.

Wounds & Cuts – niaouli oil has strong disinfectant properties, and is therefore capable of inhibiting the growth of harmful bacteria or microbes in cuts or sores. It helps to prevent infection and speed up the healing process. Mix 3 drops with 1 teaspoon of coconut oil, and massage directly over the cut twice per day.

Neroli Oil

Neroli, also known as orange blossom, is a fantastic oil for aging skin as it stimulates and promotes cell regeneration; very beneficial for use of stretch marks and scars. Its calming properties help to lift depression, ease stress and tension, reduce insomnia, and soothe nerve endings. Helps to uplift the mind and calm the senses in times of stress.

Properties: antibacterial, antidepressant, anti-inflammatory, antiseptic, antispasmodic, carminative, cicatrisant, deodorant, digestive, nervine, sedative.

Ways to Use Neroli Essential Oil

Aging Skin – neroli oil promotes the regeneration of skin cells and improves skin elasticity, making it an ideal oil to use for aging, mature skin. Mix 4 drops of the oil with 1 teaspoon of coconut oil, and massage into the face and neck. Repeat daily. Alternatively add 1-2 drops to your face cream and apply as normal.

Air Freshener – neroli oil has an exquisite natural scent widely used in the perfume industry. It therefore makes for a beautiful natural air freshener. Diffuse 4 drops and allow the aroma to fill your house. You can also place 3 drops in a saucer of warm water, and place carefully on a radiator.

Anger – neroli oil helps to deeply calm the mind and dispel feelings of anger and irritability. Place 2 drops on a tissue and inhale regularly. You can also diffuse 4 drops in a room to dispel negative feelings.

Aphrodisiac – neroli oil is used in many countries as a natural aphrodisiac. Diffuse 3 drops of the oil in a room of your choice.

Confidence – place 2 drops on a tissue, and inhale regularly. You can also diffuse 4 drops to create an aroma of confidence in the room.

Depression – dilute 3 drops in 1 tablespoon of carrier oil, and add to a warm bath. Soak for 20 minutes. Diffuse 3 drops, or place 2 drops on a tissue, and inhale regularly to help lift spirits and instil feelings of joy.

Diarrhea – mix 4 drops with 1 tablespoon of carrier oil, and massage into the abdomen and lower back. Repeat daily until symptoms ease or disappear. Neroli oil helps to relax spasms in the smooth muscle of intestines that may result in diarrhea.

Eczema – neroli oil helps to alleviate any inflammation, itching, or pain associated with eczema. Dilute 4 drops of the oil with 1 teaspoon of coconut oil, and massage into the affected area. For larger areas mix 6 drops with 1 tablespoon. Repeat daily.

Heart Palpitations – diffuse 4 drops of neroli oil, or dilute 3 drops with 1 teaspoon of carrier oil, and massage into the heart and chest area. Neroli helps to improve circulation, thus easing heart palpitations and cardiac spasms.

Insomnia – neroli's relaxing and sedative properties means it is often used to treat insomnia. Diffuse 3 drops of the oil 2 hours before bedtime, or dilute 3 drops with 1 teaspoon of coconut oil, and massage into the chest, front of the neck, and across the shoulders.

Menopause – to help with irritability and anxiety that accompany menopause, mix 6 drops of neroli oil with 2 tablespoons of carrier oil, and massage into the body. You can also dilute 5 drops in 1 tablespoon of carrier oil, and add to a warm bath, or diffuse 3 drops of the oil to dissipate any feelings of irritability from the room.

Panic Attacks – neroli oil naturally relaxes the body and helps to ease panic and fear. Diffuse 3 drops of the oil if you feel on edge. You c an also place 2 drops on a tissue and inhale regularly. Alternatively create a body oil, and massage regularly – mix 6 drops with 2 tablespoons and massage the entire body.

PMS – neroli oil is a perfect choice oil to treat PMS as it helps to reduce irritability, calm the mind, and alleviate anxiety. Diffuse 3 drops to reduce the above feelings, or dilute 4 drops with 1 tablespoon of carrier oil, and add to a warm bath.

Psoriasis – regular use of neroli oil on psoriasis yields excellent results. Skin scales are greatly reduced, resulting in softer, smoother skin. Mix 4 drops of the oil with 1 teaspoon of coconut oil, and massage into the skin. Alternatively, dilute 4 drops with 1 tablespoon of carrier oil, and add to a warm bath. Soak for 20 minutes.

Scarring – mix 3 drops of neroli oil with 1 teaspoon of coconut oil, and massage into the scar tissue twice per day. Always massage gently. Neroli oil has excellent cell regeneration properties.

Shock – neroli's gentle sedating and calming properties make it an excellent oil to use in times of shock. It allows the body and mind to relax and creates a new sense of hope. Diffuse 3 drops to dissipate feelings of shock or despair from a room. You can also add it to a warm bath by diluting 4 drops with 1 tablespoon of carrier oil.

Stress – neroli oil is a fantastic tonic for the nervous system and helps to control stress levels and panic reactions. Diffuse 3 drops of the oil in times of stress. You can also create a body spray by diluting 8 drops of the oil with 200ml of water. Place in a spray bottle, and spray around your upper body when you feel the need.

Stretch Marks – mix 5 drops of neroli oil with 1 tablespoon of coconut oil, and massage into the affected area. Repeat daily, morning and night. Neroli oil helps to both prevent and diminish the appearance of stretch marks.

Thread Veins – mix 2 drops of neroli oil with 1 teaspoon of coconut oil, and gently massage over the thread veins. Repeat twice daily. Neroli helps to diminish redness on the surface of the skin and restore elasticity to blood vessels.

Varicose Veins – neroli oil helps to improve blood circulation, making it an effective natural treatment for varicose veins. Mix 5 drops of the oil with 1 tablespoon of coconut oil, and massage into the affected limb from bottom to top. Always massage towards the direction of the heart, and never massage directly over the varicose veins.

Nutmeg Oil

Nutmeg oil is an effective anti-inflammatory and pain reliever, therefore helping with muscular aches and pains, rheumatism, and arthritis. It increases circulation, invigorates the mind, and helps to relieve indigestion and diarrhea. It encourages appetite, which is useful for those suffering with anorexia nervosa.

Properties: analgesic, antioxidant, antirheumatic, antiseptic, antispasmodic, carminative, digestive, emmenagogue, laxative, stimulant, tonic.

Ways to Use Nutmeg Essential Oil

Air Freshener – nutmeg oil has a warm, spicy, aromatic scent, making it an ideal air freshener, particularly for the winter months. Diffuse 2 drops.

Colds & Flu – nutmeg oil helps to clear congestion from the respiratory tract, easing the symptoms of colds and flu. Add 2 drops with 1 teaspoon of carrier oil, and massage into the chest.

Constipation – nutmeg oil stimulates digestion, helping to maintain regular bowel movements. Mix 3 drops with 1 teaspoon of carrier oil, and massage into the abdomen in a clockwise direction.

Coughing – nutmeg oil helps to expel mucus from the respiratory tract and also eases spasms in that area that result in coughing. Add 2 drops to a steam inhalation, or mix 3 drops with 1 teaspoon of carrier oil, and massage into the chest.

Diarrhea – nutmeg oil helps to ease contractions and spasms in the intestines, thereby reducing diarrhea. Mix 3 drops with 1 teaspoon of carrier oil, and massage into the abdomen in a clockwise direction.

Digestion – nutmeg oil acts as an overall tonic for the digestive system, ensuring the process of digestion runs smoothly. Mix 3 drops with 1 teaspoon of carrier oil, and massage into the abdomen in a clockwise direction.

Fatigue – nutmeg oil stimulates a tired mind and body, helping to overcome low energy levels and mental exhaustion. Diffuse 2 drops, or place 1 drop on a tissue, and inhale regularly throughout the day.

Indigestion – nutmeg oil stimulates the digestion of food through the digestive tract, which in turn, relieves indigestion or prevents it altogether. Mix 3 drops with 1 teaspoon of carrier oil, and massage into the abdomen in a clockwise direction.

Joint Pain – nutmeg oil has the ability to relieve joint inflammation and pain. Blend 3 drops with 1 teaspoon of carrier oil, and massage into areas of concern.

Menstrual Cramps – nutmeg oil helps to relieve menstrual cramps by reducing uterine spasms. Add 3 drops to a hot compress, and drape across the abdomen, or blend 2 drops with 1 teaspoon of carrier oil, and massage into the lower abdomen in a clockwise direction.

Muscular Aches & Pains – blend 4 drops with 1 tablespoon of carrier oil, and massage into sore muscles. Nutmeg oil has a warming action on aching muscles, which reduces pain and inflammation.

Muscle Cramps – nutmeg oil contains effective antispasmodic properties, which help to relax tight muscles and ease cramping. Mix 4 drops with 1 tablespoon of carrier oil, and massage into the affected muscle and corresponding limb.

Poor Appetite – nutmeg oil stimulates the appetite, thereby encouraging increased appetite. Mix 3 drops with 1 teaspoon of carrier oil, and massage into the abdomen in a clockwise direction.

Poor Circulation – mix 3 drops with 1 tablespoon of carrier oil, and add to a warm bath. Alternatively, mix 2 drops with 1 teaspoon of carrier oil, and massage into the feet. Nutmeg oil stimulates the blood circulation, therefore improving poor and sluggish circulation.

Rheumatism – the anti-rheumatic properties contained within nutmeg oil ease this painful disorder and reduce inflamed joints. Mix 3 drops with 1 teaspoon of carrier oil, and massage into the affected area.

Orange Oil

Orange oil is an emotionally uplifting oil helping to refresh the mind, relieve tension and stress, and promote a positive outlook. It is an effective immune system booster, protecting against infections such as colds & flu. It also acts as an excellent tonic for oily skin.

Properties: antidepressant, antiseptic, antispasmodic, carminative, digestive, sedative, stomachic, tonic.

Ways to Use Orange Essential Oil

Cellulite – orange oil helps to eliminate fat deposits and toxins from the body by increasing the frequency and quantity of urination. Mix 6 drops with 1 tablespoon of carrier oil, and firmly massage into areas of concern. Repeat daily.

Constipation – orange oil acts as a tonic for the digestive system, normalizing the peristaltic action of the intestines, therefore regulating bowel movements. Mix 4 drops with 1 teaspoon of carrier oil, and massage into the abdomen in a clockwise direction. Repeat twice per day until symptoms disappear.

Depression – orange oil helps to combat depression by encouraging feelings of joy and optimism. It uplifts the spirits and creates a positive outlook on life. Diffuse 5 drops of the oil to clear negative energy from the air.

Detox – orange oil has excellent detoxifying capabilities due to its diuretic properties and the fact that it has an invigorating effect on the lymphatic system. Dilute 7 drops of the oil in 1 tablespoon of carrier oil, and add to a warm Epsom salt bath. You can also mix 4 drops with 1 teaspoon of carrier oil, and massage into the feet.

Diarrhea – mix 4 drops with 1 teaspoon of carrier oil, and massage into the abdomen. Orange oil helps to calm the stomach and ease intestinal spasms that may give rise to diarrhea.

Fluid Retention – orange oil helps to stimulate and revitalize the lymphatic system, thereby balancing fluid retention in the body by removing excess water. Blend 8 drops with 2 tablespoons of carrier oil, and massage into the body. Alternatively, dilute 7 drops in 1 tablespoon of carrier oil, and add to a warm Epsom salt bath.

High Blood Pressure – mix 4 drops with 1 teaspoon of carrier oil, and massage over the heart center. You can also massage into the feet. Orange oil has hypotensive properties, thus helping to lower blood pressure.

Immunity – orange oil boosts the immune system, helping to protect against illnesses such as colds or flu. Mix 4 drops with 1 teaspoon of carrier oil, and massage into the feet. Alternatively, dilute 6 drops with 1 tablespoon of carrier oil, and add to a warm bath. Repeat regularly, particularly during winter months.

Indigestion – mix 4 drops with 1 teaspoon of carrier oil, and massage into the upper and lower abdomen in a clockwise direction. Orange oil promotes the secretion of digestive juices and bile in the stomach, helping to regulate digestion.

Insect Repellent – orange oil acts as a highly effective natural insect repellent. Diffuse 5 drops of the oil, or place 3 drops on a cotton ball, and leave on various surfaces around the home.

Insomnia – orange oil has a sedative effect on the mind, helping to induce sleep. Place 1 drop on your pillow before bedtime, or dilute 4 drops in 1 tablespoon of carrier oil, and add to a warm bath just before bedtime.

Nervous Tension – orange oil has a relaxing, regenerative influence on the nervous system, useful for people that tend to suffer from nervous tension or panic attacks. Diffuse 5 drops in your home, or add 15 drops to a spray bottle filled with 300ml of filtered water, and spray over the upper body during times of stress. Shake well before use.

Oily Skin – mix 4 drops with 1 teaspoon of coconut oil, and massage into the face. Orange oil helps to brighten a dull complexion and clear congested, oily skin. Repeat daily.

Poor Circulation – dilute 7 drops of orange oil in 1 tablespoon of carrier oil, and add to a warm Epsom salt bath. Orange oil stimulates blood circulation.

Positive Outlook – orange oil promotes feelings of positivity and helps to create an optimistic outlook on life. Diffuse 5 drops of the oil, or place 2 drops on a tissue, and inhale regularly.

Palmarosa Oil

With excellent skincare properties, palmarosa oil is useful for treating eczema, dermatitis, scar tissue, stretch marks, and wrinkles. It has a balancing and hydrating effect on the skin and helps to balance sebum production in both oily and dry skin. Its bactericidal properties help to clear intestinal infection. Muscle stiffness is greatly reduced with the use of palmarosa oil, as well as fever symptoms.

Properties: antibacterial, antiseptic, cytophylactic, digestive, febrifuge, stimulant, tonic.

Ways to Use Palmarosa Essential Oil

Acne Scars – over time, palmarosa oil helps to reduce scarring caused by acne due to its ability to stimulate cell regeneration. Mix 3 drops with 1 teaspoon of coconut oil, and massage over the scars 2-3 times per day.

Aging Skin – palmarosa oil helps to rehydrate the skin, regenerate healthy new cells, and tone the skin, making it a very effective oil to treat aging or mature skin. Mix 4 drops with 1 teaspoon of coconut oil, and massage into the face and neck.

Appetite – palmarosa oil stimulates the appetite and is often helpful in treating cases of anorexia nervosa. Mix 4 drops with 1 teaspoon of carrier oil, and massage into the feet or abdomen. You can also dilute 5 drops in 1 tablespoon of carrier oil, and add to a bath.

Cuts & Wounds – palmarosa oil heals cuts and wounds at a faster rate due to its excellent antiseptic and cell regeneration capabilities. Mix 3 drops with 1 teaspoon of coconut oil, and dab over the affected area twice per day.

Cystitis – dilute 5 drops in 1 tablespoon of carrier oil, and add to a sitz bath. Palmarosa oil helps to clear urinary tract infections and cools down the affected area.

Dandruff – palmarosa oil has excellent hydrating properties and helps to balance sebum production in the scalp area. Mix 6 drops with 1 tablespoon of olive or coconut oil, and massage into the scalp. Leave for 30 minutes and wash hair as normal.

Dermatitis – palmarosa oil hydrates and moisturizes dry skin conditions, and stimulates the growth of new cells. Its antiseptic properties help to prevent infection and speed up the healing process. Mix 3 drops with 1 teaspoon of coconut oil, and massage into the area of concern twice daily.

Dilated Capillaries – with regular use, palmarosa oil helps to reduce the appearance of dilated capillaries under the surface of the skin. Mix 3 drops with 1 teaspoon of coconut oil, and gently massage over capillaries twice per day.

Dry Skin – mix 4 drops with 1 teaspoon of coconut oil, and massage into the face and neck twice per day. Palmarosa oil stimulates oil production in a dry skin and helps replenish lost moisture.

Fever – palmarosa oil helps to fight fever and cools down the body temperature by encouraging perspiration. Add 4 drops to a steam inhalation, or mix 4 drops with 1 teaspoon of carrier oil, and massage into the chest area.

Healthy Digestion – mix 4 drops with 1 teaspoon of carrier oil, and massage into the abdomen in a clockwise direction. Palmarosa oil stimulates the secretion of digestive juices and ensures the proper absorption of nutrients from food.

Nail Fungus – palmarosa oil is effective at clearing fungal infections. Mix 2 drops with ½ teaspoon of coconut oil, and massage into the area of concern twice per day.

Security – palmarosa oil banishes feelings of loneliness, confusion, and vulnerability, and promotes a sense of security in an individual. Place 2 drops on a tissue, and inhale regularly, or diffuse 4 drops in your home.

Oily Skin – palmarosa oil helps to balance the production of sebum in the skin, helping to reduce oily skin and bring it under control. Mix 4 drops with 1 teaspoon of coconut oil, and massage into the face and neck twice per day.

Well Being – mix 4 drops with 1 teaspoon of carrier oil and massage into the temples, shoulders and back of the neck. Palmarosa oil induces a lovely feeling of well being and contentment.

Parsley Seed Oil

An effective diuretic, parsley seed oil helps to eliminate water retention, break down fatty deposits that cause cellulite, remove toxins from the body at a faster rate, and purify the blood. It is an excellent treatment for cystitis and can help with digestive problems such as constipation and flatulence. Parsley seed oil also contains beneficial antispasmodic properties, which help to reduce muscle spasms and menstrual cramps.

Properties: antimicrobial, antiseptic, astringent, carminative, depurative, diuretic, emmenagogue, febrifuge, hypotensive, laxative, stimulant, stomachic, tonic.

Ways to Use Parsley Seed Essential Oil

Acne – parsley seed oil contains antiseptic and antibacterial properties which help to treat pimples, clean pores, and clear up any infected blemishes. Mix 2 drops with 1 teaspoon of carrier oil, and massage into the face and neck. Leave for 20 minutes and rinse off.

Arthritis & Rheumatism – because parsley seed oil is rich in detoxifying and depurative properties, it helps to rid the body of toxins such as uric acid which can have an adverse effect on our joints. Mix 3 drops with 1 teaspoon of carrier oil, and massage into joints, or dilute 5 drops with 1 tablespoon of carrier oil, and add to a warm bath.

Bruising – parsley seed oil helps to speed up the healing of bruises as it tightens broken blood vessels under the skin's surface. Mix 2 drops with ½ teaspoon of coconut oil, and massage over the bruise twice per day.

Cellulite – the detoxifying and diuretic properties found in parsley seed oil do an excellent job at eliminating toxins and fats from the body, helping to reduce the appearance of cellulite. Mix 5 drops with 1 tablespoon of coconut oil, and firmly massage into areas of concern.

Cystitis – add 2 drops to a hot compress, and drape across the abdomen. Parsley seed oil provides relief for those suffering with cystitis.

Detox – parsley seed oil is a good oil to use when you are on a detox as it further promotes the removal of potentially harmful toxins from the body. Dilute 4 drops in 1 tablespoon of carrier oil, and add to a warm Epsom salt bath.

Digestion – parsley seed oil acts as a tonic for digestion, helping to maintain a healthy digestive tract. Mix 4 drops with 1 teaspoon of carrier oil, and massage into the abdomen in a clockwise direction.

Dilated Capillaries – parsley seed oil has a contracting effect on small blood vessels under the surface of the skin, and can therefore reduce the appearance of broken capillaries on the face when used on a regular basis. Mix 3 drops with 1 teaspoon of coconut oil, and gently massage onto capillaries twice per day.

Ear Infections – parsley seed oil benefits an ear infection by helping to reduce inflammation and pain, while also fighting the infection itself. Mix 2 drops with 1 teaspoon of coconut oil, and massage behind and below the ears. Never pour the blend in the eardrum.

Fever – parsley seed oil is an effective febrifuge, and can therefore reduce body temperature and help fight the infection that causes the fever. Diffuse 4 drops, or blend 4 drops with 1 teaspoon of carrier oil, and massage into the chest.

Fluid Retention – parsley seed oil has excellent diuretic properties, which increase the frequency of urination. This helps to rid the body of excess fluid, reducing bloating and swelling. Mix 3 drops with 1 teaspoon of carrier oil, and massage into the soles of the feet. Alternatively, dilute 4 drops in 1 tablespoon of carrier oil, and add to a warm bath.

Hemorrhoids – parsley seed oil can have a positive effect on external hemorrhoids as it helps to shrink small blood vessels under the surface of the skin. Add 2 drops to a cold compress, and hold over the affected area for 5 minutes. Alternatively, dilute 4 drops in 1 tablespoon of carrier oil, and add to a sitz bath. Soak for 20 minutes.

Irregular or Missing Periods – whether your period is irregular, or you have not menstruated in some time, parsley seed oil can stimulate the secretion of specific hormones which can promote bleeding. Mix 4 drops with 1 teaspoon of carrier oil, and massage into the abdomen in a clockwise direction.

Liver Health – parsley seed oil acts as a tonic for the liver, helping to reduce liver congestion and purify the blood. Diffuse 2 drops in your home.

Poor Circulation – parsley seed oil helps to stimulate a sluggish circulation and maintain the elasticity of blood vessels. Mix 4 drops with 1 teaspoon of carrier oil, and massage into the feet, or mix 2 drops with 1 teaspoon of carrier oil, and massage into the heart area.

Patchouli Oil

Patchouli oil is a mood uplifter, helping to relieve stress-related conditions, ease tension and anxiety, and promote an overall feeling of well being. It relieves inflammation so is useful in the treatment of dry skin conditions such as eczema, dermatitis, and psoriasis. It is also a popular insect repellent.

Properties: antidepressant, anti-inflammatory, antiseptic, aphrodisiac, astringent, cicastrisant, cytophylactic, deodorant, diuretic, febrifuge, fungicide, insecticide, sedative, stomachic.

Ways to Use Patchouli Essential Oil

Acne – patchouli oil contains antibacterial, anti-inflammatory, and antiseptic qualities, and as a result acts as an excellent treatment for acne. It helps to clear congested skin, prevent infection, and ease any inflammation around blemishes. Mix 4 drops of patchouli oil with 1 teaspoon of coconut oil, and massage into the face and neck. Repeat daily.

Athlete's Foot – due to its fungicidal properties, patchouli oil is effective at clearing up and preventing fungal infections. Mix 4 drops of the oil, and massage into the affected area, paying particular attention to in between the toes. Repeat daily.

Cholesterol – cholesterol levels can be reduced with regular use of patchouli oil due to its powerful diuretic properties. As a diuretic, patchouli oil increases urination, which helps to rid the body of waste and toxins leading to a reduction in the build-up of cholesterol.

Cracked Skin – mix 4 drops with 1 teaspoon of coconut oil, and rub in the area of cracked skin. Patchouli oil stimulates the regeneration of skin cells. Repeat twice daily.

Cuts & Sores – patchouli oil helps to dry up weeping cuts and sores, and protects them from becoming infected. Mix 2 drops with 1 teaspoon of coconut oil, and massage over the affected area twice per day. Alternatively, add 2 drops to a cold compress, and hold over the area for 5 minutes.

Dandruff – using patchouli oil as a regular treatment for dandruff, will reduce flakiness and soothe the scalp. Add 5 drops to your shampoo and wash as usual. Alternatively, mix 6 drops with 1 tablespoon of coconut oil, and massage into the scalp after shampooing the hair. Leave for 1 hour, and rinse and condition as normal.

Depression – treating depression with patchouli oil helps to induce positive feelings of happiness and hope, uplift spirits, and soothe the mind. Diffuse 5 drops of the oil, or place 2 drops on a tissue, and inhale regularly. You can also dilute 6 drops in 1 tablespoon of carrier oil, and add to a warm bath.

Healthy Hair – adding 5 drops of patchouli oil to your shampoo creates shiny, lustrous hair. You can also add 5 drops to conditioner, and leave to absorb into the hair for 20 minutes before rinsing and styling as normal.

High Blood Pressure – the use of patchouli oil results in an increase in the frequency and flow of urine, which in turn, helps to reduce high blood pressure. Dilute 5 drops with 1 tablespoon of carrier oil, and add to a warm bath. Soak for 20 minutes. Alternatively, mix 4 drops with 1 teaspoon of carrier oil, and massage into the soles of the feet.

Immune System – mix 7 drops with 2 tablespoons of carrier oil, and massage into the body, or mix 4 drops of the oil with 1 teaspoon of carrier oil, and massage into the soles of the feet. Patchouli oil acts as a tonic for the immune system, helping to strengthen and protect it.

Insect Bites – patchouli oil helps to reduce any stinging and inflammation caused by insect bites. It also helps to protect them from infection. Mix 3 drops of the oil with ½ teaspoon of coconut oil, and massage into the affected area.

Insect Repellent – the insecticidal properties of patchouli oil make it an effective oil to use when repelling insects. Diffuse 4 drops of the oil, and keep it in close proximity to you.

Mature Skin – patchouli oil helps to combat the signs of aging by regenerating new skin cells, reducing the appearance of lines and wrinkles. Mix 5 drops with 1 teaspoon of coconut oil, and massage into the face and neck.

Scar Tissue – patchouli oil facilitates rejuvenation of skin cells, making it an effective treatment for scar tissue. Mix 4 drops with 1 teaspoon of coconut oil, and gently massage into the scar twice per day.

Weight Loss – patchouli oil is said to induce the loss of appetite, helping with weight loss over time. Mix 4 drops of the oil with 1 teaspoon of carrier oil, and massage into the feet, or diffuse 4 drops in your home.

Peppermint Oil

A refreshing and uplifting oil, peppermint helps to reduce mental fatigue and improve concentration. It is a great tonic for the digestive system, helping to relieve flatulence, nausea, indigestion, and heartburn. The menthol in peppermint oil helps to clear the respiratory tract, easing the symptoms of sinus blockage, asthma, bronchitis, colds and flue, and coughs.

Properties: analgesic, antiseptic, antispasmodic, astringent, carminative, cholagogue, decongestant, emmenagogue, expectorant, febrifuge, hepatic, nervine, stimulant, sudorific, vermifuge.

Ways to Use Peppermint Essential Oil

Aching Joints – add 4 drops of peppermint oil to a hot compress, and place over the affected area for 10 minutes. Peppermint oil helps to ease painful joints and reduce any inflammation that may be present.

Awaken the Senses – add 2 drops of peppermint oil to your shower gel in the morning to stimulate and refresh the senses.

Congestion – massage 2-3 drops of peppermint oil mixed with 1 teaspoon of carrier oil into the chest area to help clear nasal congestion and sinusitis.

Coughing – add 3 drops of peppermint oil to a steam inhalation, and inhale deeply for 2-3 minutes. Take a break if you need to. The peppermint will help to clear respiratory passageways and any mucus that may be present.

Dandruff – add 5 drops of peppermint oil to shampoo and wash thoroughly. Then add 3 drops to your conditioner, massage into the scalp, leave on for 10-15 minutes, and rinse.

Energy Levels – an excellent alternative to coffee, peppermint oil gives you an energetic boost when fatigue sets in. Place 2 drops on a tissue and inhale regularly when you feel the need. Alternatively, mix 3 drops with 1 teaspoon of carrier oil, and massage into the shoulders and back of the neck.

Exercise – using peppermint oil before a workout will leave you feeling energized and motivated. Place 2 drops on a tissue, and inhale regularly before exercising. Alternatively, mix 4 drops with 1 teaspoon of carrier oil, and massage into the chest and shoulders.

Flea & Insect Repellent – add 10 drops of peppermint oil to a 200ml spray bottle filled with filtered water, and spray onto the upper and lower body to repel insects.

Focus & Concentration – diffuse 4 drops of peppermint oil to improve mental clarity.

Headaches – mix 2 drops of peppermint oil with 1 teaspoon of carrier oil, and massage into the temples and back of the neck to help relieve the pain.

Hot Flashes – during menopause, hot flashes can be an uncomfortable experience. Add 10-12 drops of peppermint oil in a 300ml spray bottle filled with filtered water, and spray over the head and upper body to cool down and refresh the senses.

Itching – to help relieve itching skin caused by a rash or sunburn, mix 4 drops of peppermint oil with 2 teaspoons of carrier oil, and massage into the affected area.

Motion Sickness – mix 3 drops of peppermint oil with 1 teaspoon of carrier oil, and massage into the abdomen in a clockwise direction. This will help to calm an upset stomach.

Mouth Rinse – add 2 drops of peppermint oil to a small amount of water, and use as a mouth rinse. Do not swallow. The peppermint leaves a refreshing, clean feeling in the mouth.

Muscular Aches & Pains – mix 5 drops of peppermint oil with 1 tablespoon of carrier oil, and massage into the affected area. Peppermint oil helps to relieve pain, inflammation, and muscular spasms.

Rodents – if you have seen any pesky little mice around your house, place 2 drops of peppermint oil on a cotton ball and leave scattered around, particularly in places where there may be small mouse holes. Be careful not to leave them in places where they can be reached by pets or children.

Smelly Feet – mix 3 drops of peppermint oil with 1 teaspoon of carrier oil, and massage into the soles of the feet. 1-2 drops of peppermint oil can also be placed inside the shoes.

Ticks – if you have the misfortune of finding a tick burrowed into your skin, place 1 drop of peppermint oil on a cotton bud and rub it around the area. This will cause the tick to poke its head out so you can remove it safely.

Tired, Sore Feet – for tired, overworked feet, add 4 drops of peppermint oil into a foot bath with relatively warm water and soak. The peppermint oil will help to reduce any swelling and relieve pain.

Toothache – to help relieve pain and soothe the muscles of the gum, place 1 drop of peppermint oil onto your toothbrush and gently clean your teeth.

Petitgrain Oil

A great stress-reliever, petitgrain oil has a calming effect on the body, helping to soothe anxiety and tension, ease a hyperactive body and mind, reduce a rapid heartbeat, calm breathing, and relax nervous spasms. It is also an effective tonic for oily skin, helping to clear excessive perspiration, while toning the skin.

Properties: antidepressant, antispasmodic, deodorant, digestive, sedative, stomachic, tonic.

Ways to Use Petitgrain Essential Oil

Acne – petitgrain oil has a cleansing effect on acne and helps to control the production of oil in the skin. Mix 3 drops with ½ teaspoon of coconut oil, and massage into the face and neck.

Addictions – petitgrain oil helps to restore emotional balance, while trying to overcome addictions. Add 10 drops to a spray mist, and lightly spray over the face when you feel the need. You can also diffuse 4 drops in your home.

Air Freshener – petitgrain oil makes for a wonderful natural air freshener due to its light, fresh, citrus scent. Diffusing 4 drops will fill your home with a beautiful fresh smell.

Anger & Bad Temper – petitgrain oil soothes the nervous system, helping to calm anyone feeling angry or bad tempered. Place 10 drops in a spray bottle filled with 300ml of filtered water, and mist lightly onto the face during times of stress.

Cuts & Wounds – petitgrain oil has excellent antiseptic properties, which help to clean cuts and wounds, preventing them from becoming infected. Mix 2 drops with ½ teaspoon of coconut oil, and massage over the area of concern twice per day.

Depression – petitgrain oil has a positive effect on our mind and emotions, helping to uplift spirits and instil feelings of happiness and joy. Diffuse 4 drops to clear the air from any negativity. You can also place 2 drops on a tissue, and inhale regularly when you are feeling down.

Insomnia – petitgrain oil helps to promote a peaceful sleep by relaxing and sedating the mind and emotions. Place 2 drops on your pillow before bedtime, or diffuse 4 drops about 15 minutes before you go to bed.

PMS – petitgrain oil's calming effect on the body helps to ease the symptoms of PMS such as irritability, restlessness, mood swings, and anxiety. Mix 4 drops with 1 teaspoon of carrier oil, and massage into the feet. You can also diffuse 4 drops to clear the air of any negativity.

Rapid Heartbeat – diffuse 5 drops to instil calm and peacefulness in your home. You can also mix 3 drops with 1 teaspoon of carrier oil, and massage over the heart area to ease a rapid heartbeat.

Vomiting – petitgrain oil eases the urge to vomit by reducing spasms in the stomach, therefore restoring balance to the digestive system. Mix 3 drops with 1 teaspoon of carrier oil, and massage into the abdomen in a clockwise direction.

Pimento Oil

Pimento oil has a deeply warming effect on the body. On an emotional level, it helps to ground the body and balance the emotions, whereas on a physical level, its warming action eases painful or stiff joints, sore muscles, and neuralgia. It is helpful at treating digestive ailments such as indigestion, nausea, intestinal cramps, and flatulence.

Properties: anesthetic, analgesic, antioxidant, antiseptic, carminative, relaxant, rubefacient, stimulant, tonic.

Ways to Use Pimento Essential Oil

Aphrodisiac – used very occasionally, pimento oil can enhance sexual desire and increase libido. Diffuse 2 drops in the bedroom.

Arthritis & Rheumatism – pimento oil possesses excellent warming capabilities and can therefore alleviate the discomfort and pain of arthritis and rheumatism. Mix 2 drops with 1 tablespoon of carrier oil, and massage into sore joints.

Coughing – pimento oil helps to calm an exhausting cough by massaging 1 drop blended with 1 teaspoon of carrier oil into the chest.

Cuts & Wounds – pimento oil protects cuts and wounds from bacterial growth and helps to ease any pain or discomfort. Add 1 drop to a cold compress, and hold over the area of concern.

Headaches – pimento oil helps to relieve the nagging pain of a headache but should only be used in small amounts. Blend 1 drop with 1 teaspoon of carrier oil, and massage into the temples and back of the neck, or diffuse 1-2 drops in your home.

Muscular Aches & Pains – pimento oil helps to ease sore muscles and also helps to alleviate muscle stiffness. Mix 2 drops with 1 tablespoon of carrier oil, and massage into the aching muscle. Alternatively, dilute 1 drop with 1 teaspoon of carrier oil, and add to a warm bath.

Poor Circulation – the warming properties contained within pimento oil help to increase blood circulation resulting in better absorption of nutrients around the body. Dilute 1 drop in 1 teaspoon of carrier oil, and add to a warm bath, or mix 2 drops with 1 teaspoon of carrier oil, and massage into the soles of the feet.

Stress – pimento oil has a warming, relaxing effect on the body and can also ease an overactive mind in times of stress. Diffuse 2 drops in your home.

Tight, Stiff Muscles – mix 2 drops with 1 tablespoon of carrier oil, and massage into stiff muscles to loosen and therefore increase mobility.

Vomiting – pimento oil gives great relief to vomiting and intestinal spasms. Mix 1 drop with 1 tablespoon of carrier oil, and massage into the abdomen in a clockwise direction.

Pine Oil

A powerful expectorant, pine oil is used to treat bronchitis, asthma, catarrh, colds and flu, coughing, and laryngitis. It has an invigorating effect on the body and mind, helping to clear mental and physical fatigue. Pine oil is effective at treating cystitis, urinary infections, and muscular pain. Its warming qualities help with arthritis and rheumatism, and also help to stimulate poor circulation.

Properties: antimicrobial, antirheumatic, antiseptic, antiviral, bactericidal, deodorant, diuretic, expectorant, insecticidal, rubefacient, tonic.

Ways to Use Pine Essential Oil

Arthritis & Rheumatism – mix 3 drops with 1 tablespoon of carrier oil and massage into painful joints. Pine oil eases the pain of arthritis and rheumatism, and also reduces inflammation around the joints.

Athlete's Foot – mix 3 drops with 1 teaspoon of coconut oil, and massage into the foot and in between the toes. Pine oil is effective at clearing the fungal infection and preventing it from spreading.

Bronchitis – pine oil is a valuable expectorant and is therefore effective at loosening phlegm and mucus from the respiratory tract, relieving bronchitis. Add 3 drops to a steam inhalation, or mix 3 drops with 1 teaspoon of carrier oil, and massage into the chest area.

Cystitis – pine oil's antiseptic and antibacterial properties help to clear urinary tract infections, particularly cystitis. It is also capable of reducing any pain and discomfort that may accompany this disorder.

Dandruff – pine oil promotes the elimination of toxins from the scalp and helps to clear dead, scaly skin. Mix 4 drops with 1 tablespoon of olive or coconut oil, and massage into the scalp. Leave for 30 minutes and wash hair as normal.

Depression – pine oil creates feelings of happiness and joy, while increasing self confidence, therefore overcoming feelings of unworthiness. It is a great oil to use for lifting the spirits. Mix 4 drops with 1 teaspoon of carrier oil, and massage into the feet, or diffuse 3 drops in your home to create a positive atmosphere.

Detox – pine oil's diuretic properties result in increased urination, which leads to the faster elimination of toxins and wastes from the body. Dilute 4 drops in 1 tablespoon of carrier oil, and add to a warm Epsom salt bath.

Mental Fatigue – pine oil helps to revitalize the nervous system to produce a clear, invigorated mind. Diffuse 3 drops in your home.

Muscular Aches & Pains – pine oil helps to ease aching muscles and reduce inflammation, particularly after exercise. Dilute 4 drops in 1 tablespoon of carrier oil, and add to a warm bath. You can also mix 4 drops with 1 tablespoon of carrier oil, and massage into sore muscles.

Sinusitis – pine oil is an excellent decongestant helping to clear mucus from the nasal passageways, allowing you to breathe more easily. Add 3 drops to a steam inhalation, or place 2 drops on a tissue, and inhale regularly.

Ravensara Oil

With excellent antiviral properties, ravensara oil is an effective treatment for cold sores, shingles, and warts. It is also often the oil of choice during colds and flu due to its strong antiviral action on the body. It is an immunostimulant, which keeps the immune system strong and supported. Ravensara oil is a great muscle relaxant and also helps to relieve muscular aches and pains. Its analgesic properties make it a beneficial oil to use for arthritis and rheumatism.

Properties: antimicrobial, antiseptic, antiviral, expectorant.

Ways to Use Ravensara Essential Oil

Aging Skin – ravensara oil contains mild antioxidant properties, which, when added to skincare, can have a positive effect on wrinkle formation. Add 2 drops to your moisturizer each morning, or mix 4 drops with 1 teaspoon of coconut oil, and massage into the face and neck.

Bacterial Infections – with powerful antimicrobial and antibacterial properties, ravensara oil is highly effective at clearing bacterial infections, both internally and externally. Mix 6 drops with 1 tablespoon of carrier oil, and add to a warm bath, or diffuse 4 drops in your home. For external skin conditions, mix 4 drops with 1 teaspoon of coconut oil, and apply over the affected area twice per day.

Bronchitis – ravensara oil is effective at clearing a congested respiratory tract by expelling mucus and phlegm build-up, therefore easing breathing. Add 4 drops to a steam inhalation, or mix 4 drops with 1 teaspoon of carrier oil, and massage into the chest.

Cold Sores – mix 1 drop of ravensara oil with 1 drop of coconut oil, and apply to the cold sore using a clean cotton swab. Repeat 2-3 times per day. Ravensara oil possesses potent antiviral capabilities and is therefore very effective at cleaning a cold sore.

Coughing – ravensara oil is particularly helpful at easing a cough as it breaks down catarrh or phlegm in the respiratory tract. It also helps to ease spasms in the chest that lead to persistent coughing. Add 3 drops to a steam inhalation, or blend 4 drops with 1 teaspoon of carrier oil, and massage into the chest.

Chronic Fatigue Syndrome – this condition can be relieved greatly by inhaling ravensara oil for about 10-15 seconds at a time. It stimulates both body and mind, increases circulation, and promotes a positive outlook.

Cuts & Wounds – mix 3 drops with 1 teaspoon of carrier oil, and apply over the area of concern twice per day. Alternatively, add 2 drops to a cold compress, and drape over the cut or wound for 30 minutes. The antiseptic properties contained within ravensara oil help to protect cuts and wounds from infection.

Depression – ravensara oil can help an individual overcome feelings of despair and sadness by invoking positive thoughts and energy. Diffuse 4 drops in the home to dispel negative energy.

Energy Levels – add 20 drops to a 300ml spray bottle filled with filtered water, and lightly mist over the upper body throughout the day. Ravensara oil boosts energy levels due to its stimulating action on the physical body.

Headaches – small quantities of ravensara oil help to ease the pain of a headache when massaged into the temples. Mix 2 drops with 1 teaspoon of carrier oil, and massage into the temples and back of the neck.

Head Lice – ravensara oil is an effective treatment against head lice, helping to destroy the infestation. Mix 6 drops with 1 tablespoon of carrier oil, and massage into the scalp. Leave for 20 minutes and rinse.

Immunity – ravensara oil is an excellent immunostimulant, helping to strengthen and support the immune system, protecting it from illness and viruses. Blend 6 drops in 1 tablespoon of oil, and add to a warm bath, or mix 4 drops with 1 teaspoon of carrier oil, and massage into the soles of the feet.

Influenza – ravensara oil is extremely effective at both preventing the onset of influenza and treating the virus at source due to its antiviral capabilities. Add 3 drops to a steam inhalation, diffuse 4 drops in your home, or mix 6 drops with 1 teaspoon of carrier oil, and add to a warm bath.

Mental Fatigue – ravensara oil acts as a mental stimulant, helping to clear fatigue and reinstate focus and concentration. Diffuse 4 drops, or mix 4 drops with 1 teaspoon of carrier oil, and massage into the soles of the feet.

Mumps & Measles – the strong antiviral action of ravensara oil makes it an extremely effective treatment for mumps, measles, or chicken pox as it destroys the virus inside the body. Mix 5 drops with 1 tablespoon of coconut oil, and dab onto affected areas. Repeat twice per day.

Muscular Aches & Pains – the powerful analgesic properties contained within ravensara oil help to ease sore, aching muscles. Mix 5 drops with 1 teaspoon of carrier oil, and massage into the affected area. Alternatively, mix 6 drops with 1 tablespoon of carrier oil, and add to a warm bath.

Nail Fungus – mix 3 drops with 1 teaspoon of coconut oil, and massage over the area of concern twice per day. Alternatively, add 3 drops to a small bowl of warm water, and soak the fingernails for 20 minutes. Ravensara oil helps to destroy and inhibit the spread of a fungal nail infection.

Shingles – mix 5 drops of ravensara oil with 1 tablespoon of coconut oil, and gently dab over areas of concern. Do not massage if too painful. Repeat twice per day to allow ravensara's excellent antiviral properties to kill the herpes zoster virus.

Sinusitis – ravensara oil helps to clear a congested nasal passageway due to its excellent decongestant capabilities. Place 2 drops on a tissue and inhale regularly when needed, or diffuse 4 drops within close proximity to you.

Tense Muscles – ravensara oil has a calming, relaxing effect on muscles. Mix 5 drops with 1 tablespoon of carrier oil, and massage into the area of concern, or dilute 6 drops with 1 tablespoon of carrier oil, and add to a warm bath.

Rose Oil

With a calming and balancing effect on the brain, rose oil helps to stimulate positive emotions and create a sense of well being. Its antiseptic and astringent properties help to treat oily, acne skin, while its anti-inflammatory properties help to reduce redness and an inflamed skin, making it an effective treatment for eczema and psoriasis.

Properties: antidepressant, antiseptic, antispasmodic, antiviral, aphrodisiac, astringent, bactericidal, cicatrisant, depurative, emmenagogue, hepatic, laxative, sedative, stomachic, tonic.

Ways to Use Rose Essential Oil

Amenorrhea (Absence of Menstruation) – rose oil stimulates the secretion of certain hormones that are responsible for starting menstruation. Mix 4 drops of the oil with 1 teaspoon of carrier oil, and massage into the lower abdomen in a clockwise direction.

Broken Capillaries – rose oil helps to contract blood vessels near the surface of the skin due to its powerful astringent properties, therefore having a diminishing effect on broken capillaries and thread veins. Mix 4 drops of the oil with 1 teaspoon of coconut oil, and gently massage over thread veins. Repeat daily.

Depression – rose oil has excellent antidepressant qualities helping to lift the spirits and invoke feelings of happiness and optimism. Diffuse 4 drops of the oil to clear negative energy in the room, or mix 3 drops with ½ teaspoon of carrier oil, and massage into the heart area. Repeat daily.

Detox – due to rose oil's depurative properties, it helps to purify the blood, therefore assisting in the removal of toxins and wastes from the circulatory and lymphatic systems. Mix 4 drops of the oil with 1 teaspoon of carrier oil, and massage into the soles of the feet. Repeat daily for 14 days.

Digestion – mix 3 drops with 1 teaspoon of carrier oil, and massage into the abdomen in a clockwise direction. Rose oil helps to promote the flow of bile, therefore facilitating the proper digestion of foods.

Dysmenorrhea (Painful Menstruation) – rose oil helps to ease the pain of menstrual cramps by reducing spasms in the uterus. Mix 4 drops of the oil with 1 teaspoon of carrier oil, and massage into the lower abdomen in a clockwise direction. Repeat several days before menstruation.

Grief – whether you are grieving over the death of a loved one or a relationship break up, rose oil possesses excellent therapeutic properties, which have an uplifting effect on the emotions. Mix 3 drops with 1 teaspoon of carrier oil, and massage into the heart area, or diffuse 4 drops in your home to dispel heavy energies.

Insomnia – place 2 drops of rose oil on your pillow before bedtime, or diffuse 4 drops in your bedroom. Rose oil contains relaxing and sedative properties, helping to calm the body and mind for a good night's sleep.

Irregular Menstruation – mix 4 drops with 1 teaspoon of carrier oil, and massage into the lower abdomen in a clockwise direction. Rose oil acts as a tonic for the uterus, helping to regulate the menstrual cycle. Repeat daily until symptoms ease.

Liver Function – rose oil acts as a tonic for the liver, boosting its strength and protecting it from infection. Mix 4 drops of the oil with 1 teaspoon of carrier oil, and massage into the soles of the feet. Repeat daily during times of illness.

Mature Skin – over time, rose oil helps to tone and lift the skin, helping to improve skin elasticity. Mix 4 drops with 1 teaspoon of coconut oil, and massage into the face and neck. Alternatively, add 1 drop to your moisturizer each day and night, and apply to your skin as normal.

Menopause – regular use of rose oil can help delay the onset of menopause, and is effective at relieving post menopausal symptoms including lack of energy, depression, mood swings, bloating, and poor circulation. Mix 4 drops of the oil in 1 teaspoon of carrier oil, and massage into the chest and heart area. Alternatively, dilute 4 drops in 1 teaspoon of carrier oil, and add to a warm bath, or regularly diffuse 4 drops in your home.

PMS – rose oil helps to relieve common symptoms of PMS including irritability, frustration, nausea, fatigue, and low moods. Diffuse 4 drops of the oil, or mix 4 drops with 1 teaspoon of carrier oil, and massage into the soles of the feet. You can also add 10 drops to a 300ml spray bottle of filtered water, and spray the upper body several times per day. Shake well before use.

Poor Circulation – dilute 4 drops of rose oil with 1 tablespoon of carrier oil, and add to a warm bath. You can also mix 3 drops with 1 teaspoon of carrier oil, and massage into the heart area. Rose oil promotes circulation and tones blood capillaries.

Scar Tissue – regular use of rose oil has a significant effect on reducing the appearance of scar tissue. Mix 2 drops with ½ teaspoon of coconut oil, and massage into the scar twice per day.

Self Esteem & Confidence – rose oil is an excellent choice for anyone with low self esteem issues. It is often called the essential oil of love, as it helps to open the heart center to receive love and strength, helping a person to love oneself and reduce feelings of fear or unworthiness. Diffuse 4 drops of the oil to clear the air, or mix 3 drops with ½ teaspoon of carrier oil, and massage into the heart area.

Semen Production – regular use of rose oil can help to increase semen production, while at the same time, easing any emotional inadequacies that might be experienced due to infertility. Dilute 4 drops of the oil in 1 teaspoon of carrier oil, and add to a warm bath. You can also diffuse 4 drops in your home, or mix 4 drops with 1 teaspoon of carrier oil, and massage into the lower abdomen. Repeat daily.

Stress & Nervous Tension – rose oil helps to comfort and soothe the nervous system, relieving symptoms of stress and nervous tension. Mix 3 drops of the oil with 1 teaspoon of carrier oil, and massage into the soles of the feet. You can also diffuse 4 drops in your home, or dilute 3 drops in 1 teaspoon of carrier oil, and add to a warm bath.

Uterine Function – rose oil possesses excellent cleansing, purifying, and regulating qualities, ensuring proper uterine function. Mix 4 drops of the oil with 1 teaspoon of carrier oil, and massage into the abdomen in a clockwise direction. You can also massage the formula into the soles of the feet.

Wrinkles – rose oil helps to smooth the appearance of fine lines and wrinkles when used regularly in any skincare regime. To create a facial oil, mix 4 drops of the oil with 1 teaspoon of coconut oil, and massage into the face and neck. Alternatively, add 2 drops to your normal moisturizer each day, and apply as normal.

Rosemary Oil

Rosemary oil is a great all round oil. It is an excellent brain tonic as it refreshes and clears the mind, increasing concentration and mental clarity. It is used to treat lack lustre hair, dandruff, bad breath, and gingivitis. It also reduces congested, oily skin, eases arthritis and rheumatism, and relieves headaches and migraines.

Properties: analgesic, antidepressant, astringent, carminative, cephalic, cholagogue, digestive, diuretic, emmenagogue, hepatic, hypertensive, nervine, rubefacient, stimulant, sudorific, tonic.

Ways to Use Rosemary Essential Oil

Aches & Pains – dilute 5 drops of rosemary oil in 1 tablespoon of carrier oil, and add to a warm bath. Rosemary oil has excellent analgesic properties, therefore helping to ease general aches and pains.

Acne – mix 4 drops of rosemary oil with 1 tablespoon of coconut oil, and gently massage into the face and neck. Leave on the skin to absorb. Rosemary oil helps to clear congested skin and eases any inflammation that may accompany this skin disorder.

Arthritis – mix 4 drops of rosemary oil together with 1 teaspoon of carrier oil, and massage into the affected area. Rosemary oil is a natural pain reliever.

Bell's Palsy – rosemary oil is a brain stimulant and therefore helps to stimulate nerve endings. Mix 2 drops of the oil with 1 teaspoon of carrier oil, and massage into the front and back of the neck, and the forehead. It can also be used on other areas affected by a stroke.

Bronchitis – rosemary oil helps to ease breathing and alleviate congestion. Add 3 drops to a steam inhalation, or mix 4 drops with 1 teaspoon of carrier oil, and massage the formula into the chest.

Cellulite – blend 5 drops of rosemary oil with 1 tablespoon of carrier oil, and massage into the affected area to help break up fat deposits and stimulate circulation.

Dandruff – mix 6 drops of rosemary oil with 1 tablespoon of coconut oil, and massage into the scalp. Leave for 30 minutes, and rinse as normal. Rosemary oil is an excellent tonic for the hair and scalp, helping to relieve dry skin disorders. Repeat 3 times per week.

Fluid Retention – rosemary oil has excellent diuretic properties and is therefore an effective way to treat fluid retention. Add 6-8 drops of rosemary oil with 1 tablespoon of carrier oil, and massage into the affected area, always ensuring that you massage upwards towards the heart. Alternatively, dilute 5 drops with 1 tablespoon of carrier oil, and add to a warm bath. Soak for 20 minutes.

Hair Growth – rosemary oil increases circulation to the scalp and is therefore an effective treatment to promote hair growth. Blend 8 drops of rosemary oil with 1 tablespoon of extra virgin olive oil, and thoroughly massage into the scalp. Leave for 30 minutes and rinse.

Headaches/Migraines – mix 2 drops of rosemary oil together with 1 teaspoon of carrier oil, and massage into the temples and back of the neck. Rosemary oil helps to alleviate the pain of a headache.

Memory Loss – diffuse 5 drops of rosemary oil in your home or office to stimulate the brain and help improve memory.

Mental Fatigue – rosemary oil is an excellent brain stimulant, helping to clear the head and improve concentration. Place 3 drops on a tissue, and inhale throughout the day when required. You can also diffuse 4 drops in your home or office.

PMS – rosemary oil has uplifting properties and is an ideal oil to use when suffering from low moods or irritability. Diffuse 5 drops of the oil, and allow the aroma to fill the room.

Puffy Skin – rosemary oil helps to reduce any puffiness or swelling of the skin. Mix 4 drops of the oil with 1 teaspoon of coconut oil, and massage into the affected area.

Sinusitis – diffuse 5 drops of the oil to help clear congestion in the nasal passageways. Alternatively, add 3 drops to a steam inhalation, and breathe deeply for 2-3 minutes.

Rosewood Oil

Also known as bois de rose, rosewood oil is fantastic to use on the face. It helps to rejuvenate and brighten the complexion, regenerate new skin cells, clear blemishes, reduce the signs of aging, and protect the skin from harmful bacteria. It also has a calming effect on the mind, instilling feelings of confidence and self esteem.

Properties: antidepressant, antiseptic, bactericide, cephalic, cytophylactic, deodorant, insecticide, stimulant.

Ways to Use Rosewood Essential Oil

Cuts & Wounds – rosewood oil has excellent healing properties for cuts and wounds. Apply 2 drops on a clean, damp gauze, and place over the area of concern for 30 minutes.

Depression – rosewood oil combats depression in a very effective way. It provokes a positive outlook on life and instils feelings of hope and optimism. Diffuse 5 drops to help lift spirits.

Emotional Imbalance – diffusing 5 drops of rosewood oil in your home has a calming effect on the mind and emotions, helping to bring about emotional stability and strength.

Fatigue – rosewood oil calms, while at the same time, has an uplifting effect on the mind and emotions. Add 10 drops to a spray bottle filled with 300ml of water, and regularly spray over the upper body. You can also place 2 drops on a tissue and inhale regularly in times in need.

Insect Repellent – rosewood oil is a highly effective insecticide which repels bugs and mosquitoes. Diffuse 5 drops in your home, or apply 3 drops to a cotton ball and leave in various places around your house.

Logical Thinking – diffuse 5 drops in your home. Rosewood oil helps to clear the head, and steady the nerves.

Mature Skin – mix 4 drops with 1 teaspoon of coconut oil, and massage into the face and neck. Alternatively, add 2 drops to your moisturizer each morning, and carry out your skincare regime as normal. Rosewood oil improves skin tone and increases skin elasticity.

Scar Tissue – rosewood oil helps to diminish the appearance of scars due to its cell regenerating properties. Mix 2 drops with ½ teaspoon of coconut oil, and gently massage over scar tissue. Repeat daily.

Stress & Tension – diffuse 5 drops to clear a tense or stressful energy in a room. Rosewood oil acts as a very good tonic for the nervous system helping to relieve symptoms of stress and tension.

Wrinkles & Fine Lines – rosewood oil helps to reduce the appearance of fine lines and wrinkles due to its regenerating effect on skin cells. Mix 4 drops with 1 teaspoon of coconut oil, and massage into the face and neck. Repeat daily.

Sandalwood Oil

A powerful anti-aging oil, sandalwood helps skin retain its moisture, calms dilated capillaries, and helps to reduce high coloring. It provides relief from inflammation, soothes tension, and helps to relieve urinary infections such as cystitis.

Properties: anti-inflammatory, antiseptic, antispasmodic, astringent, carminative, diuretic, emollient, expectorant, sedative, tonic.

Ways to Use Sandalwood Essential Oil

Acne – sandalwood oil has an antiseptic effect on blemishes, helping to speed up the healing process and protect the pimples from becoming infected. Mix 2 drops with ½ teaspoon of coconut oil and apply to each pimple. Leave to absorb into the skin. Repeat daily.

Acne Rosacea – mix 2 drops of sandalwood oil with 1 teaspoon of coconut oil, and massage into the face. Sandalwood helps to reduce high coloring and calm any redness of the skin. Repeat daily.

Bronchitis – sandalwood oil is a valuable expectorant where congestion is present. Add 3 drops to a steam inhalation, or mix 2 drops with 1 teaspoon of carrier oil and massage into the chest area.

Cold Sores – applying sandalwood oil topically over a cold sore helps to fight the infection, prevent it from spreading, and reduce inflammation around the area. Blend 1 drop of the oil with 1 drop of coconut oil, and apply directly onto the cold sore using a cotton bud.

Cystitis – sandalwood oil helps to reduce inflammation of the mucus membrane of the genito-urinary system, thereby reducing the symptoms of cystitis. Add 2 drops to a cold compress treatment, and hold over the area for 5 minutes. You can also dilute 3 drops in 1 teaspoon of carrier oil, and add to a warm sitz bath.

Diarrhea – mix 3 drops with 1 teaspoon of carrier oil, and massage into the abdomen in a clockwise direction. Sandalwood oil helps to relieve diarrhea by reducing spasms within the intestines.

Dry Hair – sandalwood oil is an excellent conditioning oil for dry, damaged hair. After shampooing, mix 4 drops with 1 tablespoon of coconut oil, and massage into the scalp and hair. Leave for 1 hour, and rinse and condition as normal.

Dry Skin – with excellent moisturizing capabilities, sandalwood oil makes a beneficial facial serum for dry skin. Mix 2 drops with 1 teaspoon of coconut oil, and massage into the face and neck. Repeat daily.

Dry, Tickly Cough – sandalwood oil helps to reduce internal spasms that cause a cough, it helps to clear any mucus build up in the respiratory tract, and soothes dry, itchy coughs. Mix 3 drops with 1 teaspoon of carrier oil, and massage into the chest area. Repeat daily until symptoms ease.

Eczema – mix 2 drops of sandalwood oil with 1 teaspoon of coconut oil, and massage into the area of concern. Sandalwood oil possesses excellent moisturizing properties, as well as having an anti-inflammatory effect on the skin.

Fever – sandalwood oil has a cooling effect on the body and also helps to reduce inflammation caused by fever. Add 3 drops with 1 teaspoon of carrier oil, and massage into the feet.

High Blood Pressure – sandalwood oil is an effective hypotensive oil and therefore has the effect of lowering high blood pressure when applied to the body. Mix 2 drops with 1 teaspoon of carrier oil and massage over the heart center.

Insect Bites – sandalwood oil helps to reduce inflammation and provide relief from insect bites and stings. Mix 2 drops with ½ teaspoon of coconut oil, and apply over the bite or sting. Repeat 2-3 times per day.

Insomnia – sandalwood oil's sedative nature calms and relaxes the nervous system, preparing the body for a peaceful night's sleep. Mix 2 drops with 1 teaspoon of carrier oil, and massage into the upper chest and back of the neck.

Memory Loss – sandalwood oil has a calming effect on the brain and helps to reduce inflammation of brain tissue. Mix 2 drops with 1 teaspoon of carrier oil, and massage into the back of the neck, or diffuse 3 drops in your home.

Muscular Cramps – sandalwood oil helps to relax muscle contractions and spasms, making it a valuable treatment for any type of muscle cramps. Mix 4 drops with 1 tablespoon of carrier oil, and massage the entire limb. Alternatively, apply a cold compress with 3 drops of sandalwood oil over the area where you feel the cramp.

Scar Tissue – sandalwood oil contains excellent cicatrisant properties, which help to speed up the healing of scar tissue. Mix 2 drops of the oil with ½ teaspoon of coconut oil, and gently massage over scar tissue. Repeat daily.

Stress & Tension – dilute 4 drops in 1 tablespoon of carrier oil, and add to a warm bath or, diffuse 3 drops in your home to clear the air. An effective sedative oil, sandalwood has a very relaxing effect, as well as being slightly uplifting.

Thread Veins – sandalwood oil helps to calm the redness of broken capillaries. Mix 2 drops with ½ teaspoon of coconut oil, and gently massage over thread veins. Repeat daily.

Vomiting – sandalwood oil helps to relieve intestinal spasms and/or inflammation, which in turn, eases nausea or vomiting. Mix 3 drops with 1 teaspoon of carrier oil, and massage into the abdomen in a clockwise direction.

Spearmint Oil

This oil is similar to peppermint oil but more gentle to use on the skin due to the lower quantities of menthol contained within it. Spearmint oil greatly benefits the digestive system by relieving problems such as constipation, flatulence, indigestion, and vomiting. It has excellent expectorant properties, which help to relieve colds and flu, coughing, asthma, and bronchitis. Feelings of stress and tension can be greatly reduced with the use of spearmint oil.

Properties: anti-inflammatory, antiseptic, antispasmodic, carminative, digestive, diuretic, emmenagogue, expectorant, febrifuge, insecticide, stimulant.

Ways to Use Spearmint Essential Oil

Acne – the antibacterial and antiseptic properties contained within spearmint oil make it an ideal treatment for acne. It also contains significantly less menthol than peppermint, making it less harsh on the skin. Mix 4 drops with 1 teaspoon of coconut oil, and massage into the face and neck.

Athlete's Foot – add 4 drops to a warm foot bath, and soak for 20 minutes. Spearmint oil helps to eliminate the fungal infection that causes this skin disorder.

Bad Breath – add 2 drops to a small amount of water, and use as a mouth wash to create a natural treatment for bad breath.

Confidence – diffusing 5 drops of spearmint oil helps to increase self confidence, overcoming shyness.

Coughing – spearmint oil contains antispasmodic properties, which help to calm a persistent cough, while its decongestant properties expel mucus from the respiratory tract. Add 3 drops to a steam inhalation, or mix 4 drops with 1 teaspoon of carrier oil, and massage into the chest.

Cuts & Wounds – the antiseptic properties contained within spearmint oil keep cuts and wounds sepsis free, while also helping to heal the skin at a faster rate.

Depression – diffusing 5 drops of spearmint oil can have a positive, uplifting effect on the senses, easing low moods and depression.

Dermatitis – dermatitis can be treated successfully using spearmint oil as it helps to reduce inflammation, prevent infection, destroy any bacteria, and accelerate the healing process. Mix 2 drops with 1 teaspoon of coconut oil, and massage into the area of concern. Repeat twice per day.

Fatigue – spearmint oil helps reduce fatigue by creating an uplifting effect on the body and mind. Diffuse 5 drops in your home, or add 15 drops to a 300ml spray bottle of filtered water, and spray over the upper body when you need an energy boost.

Gas Relief – spearmint oil helps to relax the muscles of the abdominal area, thereby allowing gas to naturally leave the body. Mix 4 drops with 1 teaspoon of carrier oil, and massage into the abdomen in a clockwise direction.

Headaches – mix 2 drops of spearmint oil with 1 teaspoon of carrier oil, and massage into the temples and back of the neck. This helps to ease the pain of a headache, particularly if it is stress related.

Household Cleaner – spearmint oil makes for an effective household cleaner due to its disinfectant qualities. Add 30 drops to a 1 liter spray bottle of filtered water, and use on kitchen and bathroom surfaces.

Indigestion – blend 3 drops with 1 teaspoon of carrier oil, and massage into the abdomen in a clockwise direction. Spearmint oil relieves the discomfort of indigestion.

Insect Repellent – spearmint oil acts as an effective insect repellent, both on the body and in a diffuser. Mix 4 drops with 1 teaspoon of carrier oil, and massage into ankles, shoulders, elbows, and knees, or diffuse 5 drops within close proximity to you.

Irregular Periods – spearmint oil promotes the secretion of estrogen, a hormone which helps to ensure regular menstruation. Mix 4 drops with 1 teaspoon of carrier oil, and massage into the lower abdomen.

Muscle Strain – mix 5 drops with 1 tablespoon of carrier oil, and massage into the aching muscle and corresponding limb. Spearmint oil helps to ease muscle strain, including any cramping associated with this condition.

Sinusitis – spearmint oil acts as a decongestant, helping to clear nasal passageways and ease breathing. Mix 4 drops with 1 teaspoon of carrier oil, and massage into the sides of the nose, behind the ears, and back of the neck.

Stomach Cramps – spearmint oil has a relaxing effect on spasms within the abdominal region that cause cramping. Mix 4 drops with 1 teaspoon of carrier oil, and massage into the abdomen in a clockwise direction.

Stress & Tension – spearmint oil promotes feelings of relaxation, and can reduce mental pressure. Place 2 drops on a tissue, and inhale regularly, or blend 4 drops with 1 teaspoon, and massage into the chest area.

Vomiting – spearmint oil eases vomiting by reducing spasms in the abdominal area and intestines. Mix 3 drops with 1 teaspoon of carrier oil, and massage into the abdomen in a clockwise direction.

Spikenard Oil

Spikenard oil is a great stress reliever and therefore helps to ease migraines, nervous tension, neck pain, restlessness, and insomnia. It has a rejuvenating effect on mature skin, helping to soften the appearance of fine lines and wrinkles. Spikenard oil helps to soothe the skin and is effective when used on rashes, skin allergies, minor burns, and psoriasis.

Properties: antibacterial, anti-inflammatory, deodorant, diuretic, fungicidal, laxative, sedative, tonic.

Ways to Use Spikenard Essential Oil

Athlete's Foot – spikenard oil contains effective fungicidal properties which help to destroy the fungus that causes athlete's foot. Add 3 drops to a warm foot bath, and soak feet for 20 minutes.

Bacterial Infections – spikenard oil can be applied to cuts or wounds to protect them from infection and is also effective when applied to bacterial skin infections such as boils, impetigo, or folliculitis. Mix 2 drops with ½ teaspoon of coconut oil, and gently massage over the affected area. Repeat twice per day.

Cellulite – spikenard oil stimulates the circulation of blood and lymph, helping with the speedier removal of toxins and wastes from the body. Mix 5 drops with 1 tablespoon of coconut oil, and firmly massage into areas of concern.

Constipation – mix 4 drops with 1 teaspoon of carrier oil, and massage into the abdomen in a clockwise direction. Spikenard oil has a laxative effect on the body and can help anyone suffering from constipation.

Itching – spikenard oil has a calming, soothing effect on itchy skin and helps to reduce any inflammation that may be present. Add 10 drops to a 300ml spray bottle of filtered water, and spray on affected areas regularly. Alternatively, mix 8 drops with 2 tablespoons of coconut oil, and massage the entire body.

Mature Skin – spikenard oil has excellent skin regeneration properties, helping to produce new skin cells, and maintain a healthy, youthful appearance. Mix 3 drops with 1 teaspoon of coconut oil, and massage into the face and neck.

Meditation – spikenard oil helps to ground a person, both emotionally and spiritually. It is therefore a beneficial oil to use during meditation. Diffuse 4 drops.

Nervous Tension – diffuse 4 drops, or mix 4 drops with 1 teaspoon of carrier oil, and massage into the feet. The sedative action of spikenard oil can help relieve nervous tension and stress.

Psoriasis – spikenard oil has skin rejuvenating properties, which help to produce new healthy skin cells, therefore replacing dry, flaky skin. Mix 3 drops with 1 teaspoon of coconut oil, and massage into the affected area. Repeat daily.

Rashes – mix 5 drops with 1 tablespoon of coconut oil, and massage into the area of concern. Spikenard oil helps to reduce an inflamed skin, soothe any itching, and prevents any infection from taking place.

Spruce Oil

Acting as a tonic for the body as a whole, spruce oil stimulates and strengthens the immune system, therefore protecting against viruses and infections. It also increases circulation, relieves inflammation around painful joints and muscles, helps to expel mucus during colds, eases coughing, and relieves the pain of sciatica. Spruce oil has a balancing effect on the emotions and can help boost energy levels.

Properties: antimicrobial, antiseptic, astringent, diaphoretic, diuretic, expectorant, nervine, rubefacient, tonic.

Ways to Use Spruce Essential Oil

Aching Joints – spruce oil relieves inflammation and eases the pain of joints. Mix 3 drops with 1 teaspoon of carrier oil, and massage into areas of concern. Alternatively, add 3 drops to a hot compress, and drape over painful joints.

Acne – acne can benefit from the astringent, antiseptic, and antimicrobial actions of spruce oil. Mix 3 drops with 1 teaspoon of coconut oil, and massage into the face and neck.

Aging Skin – spruce oil has excellent cell regenerating properties and helps to improve skin tone with regular use. Add 2 drops to your moisturizer each morning, or mix 3 drops with 1 teaspoon of carrier oil and use as a facial oil.

Athlete's Foot – spruce oil is an effective treatment for fungal infections of the skin such as athlete's foot. It helps to relieve itching and inflammation, and prevents the infection from spreading. Add 3 drops to a warm foot bath and soak for 20 minutes. Follow up with a foot lotion using a blend of 3 drops of spruce oil mixed with 1 teaspoon of coconut oil.

Bronchitis – mix 3 drops with 1 teaspoon of carrier oil, and massage into the chest area. Alternatively, add 3 drops to a steam inhalation. Spruce oil helps to dispel mucus, and clear respiratory passageways.

Carpel Tunnel Syndrome – mix 3 drops of spruce oil with ½ teaspoon of carrier oil and massage over the area. Alternatively, add 3 drops to a hot compress, and wrap around the area for 20 minutes. Spruce oil helps to reduce inflammation and relieve any pain or discomfort.

Cellulite – blend 5 drops with 1 tablespoon of coconut oil, and firmly massage into areas of concern. Spruce oil encourages the removal of wastes and toxins from the body, helping to reduce the appearance of cellulite over time.

Coughing – spruce oil eases coughing by driving out excess mucus. Add 3 drops to a steam inhalation, or mix 3 drops with 1 teaspoon of carrier oil, and massage into the chest area.

Fatigue – diffusing 4 drops of spruce oil helps to energize a fatigued mind, encouraging a fresher outlook and boosting energy levels.

Hormonal Imbalance – spruce oil helps to regulate hormones, creating a balanced endocrine system. Mix 4 drops with 1 teaspoon of carrier oil, and massage into the feet.

Immunity – spruce oil stimulates the immune system, keeping it strong and supported. Mix 4 drops with 1 teaspoon of carrier oil, and massage into the feet.

Nail Fungus – spruce oil is effective at treating nail fungus, helping to clear the infection and prevent it from multiplying. Mix 2 drops with ½ teaspoon of coconut oil, and massage over the area of concern twice per day.

Open Pores – spruce oil's excellent astringent properties make it a beneficial oil to use to tighten and tone pores. Mix 2 drops with ½ teaspoon of coconut oil, and massage over areas of concern. Alternatively, add 2 drops to a barely cold compress and drape over the face for 5 minutes. Ensure you can breathe properly.

Poor Circulation – spruce oil helps to stimulate a slow, sluggish circulation, which in turn, helps to improve nutrient absorption around the body. Mix 3 drops with 1 teaspoon of coconut oil, and massage into the feet, or dilute 5 drops in 1 tablespoon of carrier oil, and add to a warm bath.

Psoriasis – mix 3 drops with 1 teaspoon of coconut oil, and massage over the area of skin suffering from psoriasis. Spruce oil helps to reduce inflammation that can sometimes accompany this skin disorder, and also helps to speed up the healing process.

St. John's Wort Oil

St. John's Wort oil acts as an effective antidepressant, helping to uplift the spirits and instil feelings of hope and happiness. It has an overall calming effect on the nervous system, and it can help to ease the pain of arthritis, sciatica, menstrual cramps, and overworked muscles. It is a beneficial oil to use during PMS, helping to alleviate low moods, irritability, anger, and frustration. It can also promote a peaceful night's sleep.

Properties: analgesic, antibacterial, antidepressant, antiseptic, antiviral, nervine.

Ways to Use St. John's Wort Essential Oil

Bruising – mix 2 drops of St. John's wort oil, and massage gently over the bruise to help reduce swelling and speed up the healing process.

Depression – St John's wort helps to relieve depression. It eases mood swings, instils feelings of happiness, and helps to boost energy levels. Diffuse 3 drops, or place 2 drops on a tissue and inhale regularly.

Hemorrhoids – apply a cold compress with 3 drops of St. John's wort oil to help reduce inflamed hemorrhoids, and relieve pain.

Insect Bites & Stings – St. John's wort oil helps to reduce swelling around bites or stings, and also acts as an antiseptic to keep the area clean and free from infection. Mix 2 drops with ½ teaspoon of carrier oil, and dab over the area of concern twice per day.

Muscular Aches & Pains – blend 4 drops of St. John's wort with 1 tablespoon of carrier oil, and massage into sore, aching muscles to provide relief after exercise or over-exertion.

Neuralgia – the anti-inflammatory and pain relieving properties contained within St. John's wort can help to ease neuralgia. Mix 4 drops with 1 teaspoon of carrier oil, and massage into the feet. You can also mix 2 drops with ½ teaspoon of carrier oil, and gently massage over the area of concern.

PMS – St. John's wort oil is useful to use during PMS as it helps to alleviate low moods, restlessness, and anxiety. Mix 4 drops with 1 teaspoon of carrier oil, and massage into the feet, or diffuse 3 drops in your home.

Sciatica – St. John's wort has a sedative effect on nerves and helps to reduce nerve inflammation. Mix 4 drops with 1 tablespoon of carrier oil, and massage into the leg and buttock. You can also dilute 4 drops in 1 tablespoon of carrier oil, and add to a warm bath.

Sunburn – St. John's wort has antiseptic and healing properties which help to soothe sunburn skin and prevent any blisters from becoming infected. Mix 3 drops with 1 tablespoon of coconut oil and gently massage over the area. Alternatively, add 2 drops to a cold compress and drape over the sunburn.

Swollen Joints – mix 4 drops with 1 teaspoon of carrier oil, and massage into painful joints. St. John's wort oil contain excellent anti-inflammatory and pain relieving properties, which help to reduce swelling around the joints and easy any pain.

Tangerine Oil

Tangerine oil is a citrus oil which helps to stimulate blood circulation, encourage the removal of toxins from the body, reduce the appearance of cellulite, and eliminate water retention. Tangerine oil has a tonic effect on the digestive system, helping with indigestion, flatulence, and diarrhea. It is a soothing oil, promoting calm and relaxation.

Properties: antiseptic, antimicrobial, antispasmodic, carminative, cytophylactic, digestive, depurative, diuretic, sedative, stomachic, tonic,

Ways to Use Tangerine Essential Oil

Air Freshener – the beautiful fresh, citrus scent that comes from tangerine oil makes it an effective air freshener. Diffuse 4 drops in your home.

Asthma – tangerine oil can help to calm spasms in the respiratory tract, which eases troubled or difficult breathing. Mix 3 drops with 1 teaspoon of carrier oil, and massage into the chest area.

Bacterial Infection – tangerine oil has a positive effect on bacterial infections, helping to kill the bacteria and speed up the healing process. Mix 2 drops with ½ teaspoon of coconut oil, and dab over the area twice per day.

Cellulite – tangerine oil helps to break up fat deposits under the surface of the skin that cause cellulite. Mix 5 drops with 1 tablespoon of coconut oil, and firmly massage into the area of concern.

Constipation – tangerine oil has a mild laxative effect on the body. Mix 3 drops with 1 teaspoon of carrier oil, and massage into the abdomen in a clockwise direction.

Cuts & Wounds – tangerine oil contains excellent antiseptic properties and when used on cuts and wounds, it helps to kill any bacterial infection and prevent it from spreading. Mix 2 drops with ½ teaspoon of coconut oil, and dab over the area of concern twice per day.

Dandruff – tangerine oil is an effective oil to use for dandruff as it helps to ease dry, flaking skin due to its emollient properties. Blend 8 drops with 2 tablespoons of olive oil, and massage into the scalp. Leave for 30 minutes and wash hair as normal. You can also add 4 drops to 1 ounce of shampoo each time you wash your hair.

Detox – tangerine oil possesses powerful depurative and diuretic properties, therefore helping to rid the body of toxic waste by purifying and refreshing the blood. Mix 3 drops with 1 teaspoon of carrier oil, and massage into the feet, or dilute 6 drops in 1 tablespoon of carrier oil, and add to an Epsom salt bath.

Diarrhea – mix 4 drops of tangerine oil with 1 teaspoon of carrier oil, and massage into the abdomen in a clockwise direction. Tangerine oil reduces spasms in the stomach and intestines, inducing relaxation in the digestive system.

Digestion – tangerine oil acts as a tonic for the digestive system, therefore helping to maintain healthy digestion. Mix 4 drops with 1 teaspoon of carrier oil, and massage into the abdomen in a clockwise direction.

Energy Levels – place 2 drops on a tissue, and inhale regularly when needed, or add 15 drops to a 300ml spray bottle filled with filtered water, and mist over the upper body throughout the day.

Fluid Retention – dilute 6 drops with 1 tablespoon of carrier oil, and add to a warm bath, or mix 4 drops with 1 teaspoon of carrier oil, and massage into the feet. Tangerine oil acts as a diuretic, increasing the frequency and quantity of urination thereby helping to relieve excess water retention from the body at a faster rate.

Irritability – diffuse 3 drops, or place 2 drops on a tissue, and inhale regularly to reduce irritability and induce a centering, calming effect.

Lymphatic Tonic – tangerine oil helps to relieve a decongested lymphatic system by encouraging toxic waste elimination. Mix 8 drops with 2 tablespoons of coconut oil, and massage the entire body, always in the direction of the heart.

Poor Circulation – tangerine oil stimulates blood circulation, improving the transport of oxygen and nutrients around the body. Dilute 6 drops in 1 tablespoon of carrier oil, and add to a warm bath. Alternatively, mix 3 drops with 1 teaspoon of carrier oil, and massage over the heart center.

Tea Tree Oil

Tea tree oil contains an array of antiviral and antifungal benefits making it a potent healer. It helps to treat cold sores, athlete's foot, warts, verrucae, acne, dandruff, insect bites, thrush, cystitis, flu, colds, head lice, and burns. Tea tree oil can be applied neat on the skin.

Properties: antibacterial, antimicrobial, antifungal, antiseptic, cicatrisant, expectorant, fungicide, immunostimulant, insecticide, stimulant, sudorific.

Ways to Use Tea Tree Essential Oil

Arthritis – mix 5 drops of tea tree oil with 1 tablespoon of carrier oil, and massage into the affected area. Repeat when needed. Tea tree oil will help to relieve pain and reduce any inflammation that may accompany this skeletal disorder.

Athlete's Foot – tea tree oil's strong antifungal properties make it a valuable oil when it comes to athlete's foot. Mix 8 drops of tea tree oil with 1 teaspoon of carrier oil, and massage into the feet and toes. Repeat twice per day.

Bacterial Infections – bacterial infections can be effectively treated by mixing 5 drops of tea tree oil with 1 teaspoon of carrier oil and massaged into the soles of the feet. For specific bacterial skin disorders, mix 2 drops of tea tree oil with 1 teaspoon of coconut oil, and massage into the area of concern twice per day.

Bladder Infections – add a dilution of 6 drops of tea tree oil with 1 tablespoon of carrier oil, and add to a warm sitz bath. Sit for 20 minutes allowing the oils to absorb into the skin. Alternatively, add 4 drops to a hot compress, and drape across the abdomen to help relieve a bladder infection.

Blisters & Boils – apply 1 drop of tea tree oil directly on the blister or boil to prevent or minimize infection. Repeat 2-3 times per day.

Chapped Lips – add 1 or 2 drops to your lip balm, and apply to lips several times per day. Repeat daily to minimize dryness and prevent infection.

Chicken Pox – blend 10 drops of tea tree oil with 3 tablespoons of coconut oil, and massage into the skin. The strong virus-fighting capabilities of tea tree oil help to speed the healing of chicken pox, while also minimizing the risk of scarring.

Cold Sores – using a cotton swab, apply 1 drop of tea tree oil directly over the cold sore. Repeat 2-3 times per day. Tea tree oil possesses powerful antiviral properties, and as a result, can kill the virus that causes herpes simplex.

Coughing – add 4 drops of tea tree oil to a steam inhalation, or mix 3 drops with 1 teaspoon of carrier oil, and massage into the chest area. Tea tree oil helps to reduce inflamed air passageways and also promotes sweating so it can help reduce a fever.

Dandruff – dilute 10 drops of tea tree in 1 tablespoon of olive oil, and massage into the scalp. You can also add 6 drops to your shampoo, and wash hair thoroughly. Tea tree oil is an effective dandruff treatment as it helps to clear flaky skin and replenish lost moisture in the scalp.

Eczema – tea tree oil's antiseptic and anti-inflammatory properties make it an effective treatment for eczema. Mix 5 drops of tea tree oil with 1 tablespoon of carrier oil, and massage into the affected area. Repeat daily.

Garbage Freshener – add 2 drops of tea tree oil to the bottom of your garbage disposer to kill any germs or bacteria that may be present, and to create a fresh scent.

Gingivitis – mix 1 teaspoon of aloe vera gel with 3 drops of tea tree oil, and rub the mixture into the gums. Do not swallow. Alternatively, create a healing mouthwash by adding 2 drops of tea tree oil to 4 tablespoons of water, and use as a mouth wash.

Gout – massage 6 drops of tea tree oil mixed with 1 teaspoon of coconut oil into the affected area, and repeat daily until symptoms ease. Tea tree oil helps to relieve any pain and discomfort in the joints.

Head Lice – mix 15 drops of tea tree oil with 1 tablespoon of carrier oil, and massage into the scalp. Leave on for 30 minutes. Alternatively, add 10 drops to 1 ounce of shampoo and thoroughly wash the hair. Repeat 2-3 times per week until symptoms subside. Tea tree oil's strong antimicrobial properties can successfully alleviate an infestation of head lice, keeping the scalp healthy.

Immune System – tea tree oil is a powerful immuno-stimulant thus helping the body to recover from illness more quickly. It also strengthens the body to prevent illness from taking place in the first instance. Mix 8 drops of tea tree oil with 2 tablespoons of carrier oil, and massage into the body.

Insect Bites & Stings – mix 3 drops of tea tree oil with 1 teaspoon of coconut oil, and apply to the bite and surrounding tissue 3-4 times per day. This will help to relieve itching, stinging, and inflammation.

Insect Repellent – place 15 drops of tea tree oil into a 300ml spray bottle of filtered water, and spray onto ankles, knees, elbows, shoulders, and lower back. Carry out this treatment in the evening only.

Muscular Aches & Pains – blend 8 drops of tea tree oil with 1 tablespoon of carrier oil, and add to a warm bath. Soak for 20 minutes. Tea tree oil helps to reduce inflammation and ease aching muscles.

Nail Fungus – tea tree oil is a strong fungicidal so it can help clear any fungal infection present on the nail. Apply 1-2 drops of the oil on the nail, and leave to absorb into the skin. Repeat daily.

Pimples – using a cotton swab, apply 1 drop of tea tree oil directly on the pimple. Tea tree has excellent antibacterial properties, therefore helping to clear any infection.

Psoriasis – to help relieve itching and inflammation, soothe the skin, and promote healing, blend 6-8 drops of tea tree oil with 1 tablespoon of carrier oil, and add to a warm bath. Soak for 20 minutes.

Shingles – mix 8 drops of tea tree oil together with 1 tablespoon of carrier oil, and massage into the affected area. Tea tree oil helps to relieve inflammation, alleviate pain and itching, and kill the viral infection inside the body.

Sunburn – to soothe any stinging or itching from sunburn, mix 6 drops of tea tree oil with 1 tablespoon of cooled aloe vera gel, and gently massage into the affected area. Alternatively, add 4 drops to a cold compress, and drape across the sunburn.

Surface Cleaner – add 20 drops of tea tree oil in a 500ml spray bottle of water, and spray on kitchen and bathroom surfaces to help kill germs and prevent the spread of bacteria. Shake well before use.

Ticks – apply 2 drops of tea tree oil directly over the tick and wait for 2 minutes. It will loosen the tick making it easier to carefully remove it. The tea tree oil will also minimize any infection in the area.

Toothbrush – disinfect your toothbrush by applying 1 drop to the head of the toothbrush once per week.

Warts or Verrucae – tea tree oil has effective antiviral properties, thus making it the oil of choice for use on warts or verrucae. Simply apply 2 drops of tea tree oil directly onto the wart or verruca using a clean cotton swab. Repeat 2-3 times per day.

Thyme Oil

Thyme oil has excellent expectorant properties and is therefore valuable in treating respiratory disorders such as bronchitis, sinusitis, colds and flu, coughing, and asthma. It helps to treat arthritis, rheumatism, and general joint pain due to its warming action on the body. It also promotes focus and concentration, helping to relieve mental exhaustion. Thyme oil helps with blood circulation and can increases low blood pressure.

Properties: antirheumatic, antiseptic, antispasmodic, bactericide, carminative, cicatrisant, diuretic, emmenagogue, expectorant, insecticide, stimulant, tonic, vermifuge.

Ways to Use Thyme Essential Oil

Acne – mix 3 drops with ½ teaspoon of coconut oil, and massage over open pores and blemishes. The antibacterial properties in thyme oil will protect blemishes from becoming infected and help to heal the skin at a faster rate.

Arthritis – thyme oil's warming properties help to relieve pain and discomfort caused by arthritis or rheumatism. Mix 3 drops with 1 teaspoon of carrier oil, and gently massage over painful joints.

Athlete's Foot – thyme oil has excellent anti-fungal properties, helping to clear the infection that causes athlete's foot. It also prevents the infection from spreading. Mix 2 drops with 1 teaspoon of coconut oil, and gently rub over the infection, making sure to massage in between the toes.

Blood Clots – mix 3 drops of thyme oil with 1 teaspoon of carrier oil, and massage into the soles of the feet. Thyme oil stimulates a sluggish circulation.

Bronchitis – thyme oil helps to loosen and clear mucus build up from the airways, easing the symptoms of arthritis. Add 3 drops to a steam inhalation, or mix 3 drops with 1 teaspoon of carrier oil, and massage into the chest area.

Cellulite – mix 4 drops of thyme oil with 1 tablespoon of coconut oil, and massage into areas of concern. Thyme oil helps to eliminate excess fluid and break up fat deposits, helping to reduce the appearance of cellulite.

Cold Sores – thyme oil helps to keep cold sores infection-free and prevent them from spreading. Add 1 drop of thyme oil and 1 drop of coconut oil on a cotton bud, and gently pat the cold sore. Repeat twice per day.

Cuts & Sores – thyme oil helps to keep wounds, cuts and, sores clean and infection-free. Mix 2 drops with 1 teaspoon of coconut oil, and massage over the affected area twice daily.

Cystitis – dilute 4 drops with 1 tablespoon of carrier oil, and add to a warm sitz bath. You can also place 2 drops on a cold compress, and hold over the area of concern for 5 minutes. The antiseptic properties of thyme oil make it an ideal treatment for cystitis.

Detox – using thyme oil helps to rid the body of toxins, salts, and wastes that build up in the body's tissues over time. Dilute 4 drops with 1 tablespoon of carrier oil and add to a warm Epsom salt bath.

Digestion – thyme oil helps to improve a sluggish digestion. Mix 3 drops with 1 teaspoon of carrier oil, and massage into the abdomen in a clockwise direction.

Insect Bites & Stings – thyme oil safeguards bites and stings against infections and helps to keep the wounds clean. Mix 2 drops of the oil with 1 teaspoon of coconut oil, and massage over the area of concern twice per day.

Immune System – thyme oil possesses potent antiseptic and antibacterial properties, and therefore acts as a tonic for the immune system, keeping it healthy and strong. Mix 3 drops with 1 teaspoon of carrier oil and massage into the feet.

Irregular Periods – mix 3 drops with 1 teaspoon of carrier oil, and massage into the abdomen in a clockwise direction. Thyme oil helps to stimulate menstruation.

Low Blood Pressure – thyme oil stimulates the circulation and relaxes blood vessels, thereby helping to raise low blood pressure. Mix 3 drops of oil with 1 teaspoon of carrier oil and massage into the feet or heart area.

Mental Clarity – thyme oil promotes focus and concentration, helping to clear and invigorate the mind. Diffuse 4 drops, or place 2 drops on a tissue and inhale regularly.

Muscular Aches & Pains – aches and pains caused by over exercising or sporting injuries can be eased with the use of a thyme oil blend. Mix 4 drops with 1 tablespoon of carrier oil and massage into the painful area. You can also dilute 4 drops with 1 tablespoon of carrier oil and add to a warm bath.

Poor Circulation – dilute 4 drops in 1 tablespoon of carrier oil and add to a warm bath, followed immediately by a cool shower for 10 – 15 seconds. You can also mix 4 drops with 1 teaspoon of carrier oil and massage into the feet.

Valerian Oil

A very calming oil, valerian oil helps to relieve insomnia by promoting a restful night's sleep. It soothes tension, eases headaches, and has a grounding effect on over active minds. It promotes emotional balance and is a magnificent relaxing oil to use during times of stress.

Properties: antibacterial, antispasmodic, carminative, diuretic, sedative, stomachic.

Ways to Use Valerian Essential Oil

Arthritis & Rheumatism – valerian oil helps to reduce pain and inflammation associated with arthritis and rheumatism. Add 3 drops to a hot compress, and drape over aching joints.

Headaches/Migraines – blend 2 drops with ½ teaspoon of carrier oil, and massage into the temples and back of the neck. Valerian oil has a calming effect on the nervous system, which in turn, eases the pain from a headache or migraine.

Heart Palpitations – valerian oil's sedative effect on the parasympathetic nervous system helps to ease breathing and reduce an over-rapid heartbeat. Mix 3 drops with 1 teaspoon of carrier oil, and massage into the heart area.

Hyperactivity – diffuse 3 drops, or mix 3 drops with 1 teaspoon of carrier oil, and massage into the chest and across the shoulders. Valerian oil has the ability to reduce excitability, restlessness, and hyperactivity.

Insomnia – valerian oil is an effective sedative, helping to induce a restful night's sleep. Diffuse 3 drops 15 minutes before bedtime, or mix 3 drops with 1 teaspoon of carrier oil, and massage into the feet.

Meditation – valerian oil has a very calming and grounding effect on the mind and is therefore a beneficial oil to use while meditating. Diffuse 4 drops in your home.

Menstrual Cramps – valerian oil contains strong antispasmodic properties which help to soothe cramping of the uterine muscles. Mix 4 drops with 1 teaspoon of carrier oil, and massage into the lower abdomen in a clockwise direction.

Muscle Spasms – valerian oil helps to relax muscle spasms due to its antispasmodic capabilities. Mix 4 drops with 1 teaspoon of carrier oil, and massage into the area of concern.

Nervous Tension – valerian oil possesses soothing and relaxing properties, which help to settle nerves during times of stress or tension. Mix 3 drops with 1 teaspoon of carrier oil, and massage into the chest and across the shoulders. You can also dilute 4 drops in 1 tablespoon of carrier oil, and add to a warm bath.

Shock – valerian oil has a soothing effect on the parasympathetic nervous system and can therefore calm the body and mind after shock. Place 2 drops on a tissue and inhale regularly, or diffuse 3 drops in your home.

Vetiver Oil

This is a wonderful oil for promoting an overall sense of calm in both body and mind, as it helps to ease feelings of irritability, anger, and frustration. Vetiver oil is a great nourishing oil for the skin, helping to reduce fine lines and wrinkles, and reduce the appearance of stretch marks. It soothes aching muscles and joints, and also helps to relieve the pain of menstrual cramps.

Properties: analgesic, antibacterial, anti-inflammatory, antimicrobial, antiseptic, antispasmodic, depurative, emmenagogue, nervine, sedative, tonic, vermifuge, vulnerary.

Ways to Use Vetiver Essential Oil

Acne Scars – vetiver oil promotes the growth of new skin cells and therefore helps to fade acne scars when used regularly. Mix 3 drops with 1 teaspoon of carrier oil, and massage into the face and neck.

Aphrodisiac – vetiver oil is often used as an aphrodisiac to stimulate arousal and sexual desire. Diffuse 4 drops, or mix 4 drops with 1 teaspoon of carrier oil and massage into the feet.

Arthritis & Rheumatism – vetiver oil is a mild rubefacient, which is beneficial at relieving painful and stiff joints due to its warming capabilities. Mix 4 drops with 1 teaspoon of carrier oil, and massage into areas of concern.

Cuts & Wounds – vetiver oil has excellent antiseptic properties and is a great choice for treating cuts and wounds as it helps to protect from infection. Mix 3 drops with 1 teaspoon of coconut oil, and gently apply the blend to the area of concern twice daily.

Emotional Imbalance – vetiver oil helps to balance the emotions after times of shock, worry, or grief. Diffuse 5 drops, or add 15 drops to a 300ml spray mist, and lightly spray on the face at regular intervals throughout the day.

Gout – vetiver oil has powerful anti-inflammatory properties, providing relief to those suffering from gout. Mix 4 drops with 1 tablespoon of carrier oil, and massage into the area of concern in an upwards direction towards the heart.

Insomnia – place 2 drops on your pillow just before you go to bed, or diffuse 4 drops 15 minutes before bedtime. Vetiver oil acts as a sedative for the nervous system, helping to promote a restful night's sleep.

Mature Skin – vetiver oil has a rejuvenating effect on mature skin as it helps to strengthen the skin's connective tissue, therefore increasing elasticity and muscle tone. Mix 4 drops with 1 teaspoon of coconut oil, and massage into the face and neck.

Menopause – vetiver oil regulates the secretion of estrogen and progesterone, normalizing hormonal imbalance in the body, therefore helping to relieve the symptoms of menopause. Dilute 5 drops in 1 tablespoon of carrier oil and add to a warm bath. You can also add 10 drops to a 300ml spray mist, and spray over the upper body when required.

Nervous Disorders – nervous disorders such as Parkinson's disease and panic attacks can be eased by using vetiver oil due to its calming and relaxing effect on the nerves. Diffuse 5 drops in the home.

Nervous Tension & Anxiety – vetiver oil has a calming effect on the central nervous system, restoring balance to both body and mind in times of stress. Diffuse 5 drops, or add 10 drops to a 300ml spray mist, and lightly spray on the face when required.

PMS – diffuse 4 drops, or mix 4 drops with 1 teaspoon of carrier oil, and massage into the chest and across the shoulders. Vetiver oil helps to relieve the symptoms of PMS due to its regulating capabilities on the female hormones, estrogen and progesterone.

Poor Circulation – vetiver oil increases blood flow by expanding and dilating blood vessels, helping to transport more oxygen and nutrients around the body. Mix 4 drops with 1 teaspoon of carrier oil, and massage over the heart area.

Oily Skin – mix 3 drops with 1 teaspoon of coconut oil, and massage into the face and neck. Vetiver oil helps to balance oil production in the skin, which normalizes oily skin.

Stretch Marks – due to vetiver oil's skin regeneration properties, it is a beneficial oil for treating stretch marks. Mix 4 drops with 1 teaspoon of coconut oil, and massage into the area of concern. Repeat regularly.

Yarrow Oil

Yarrow oil is a particularly beneficial oil to use for treating allergies, minor burns, inflammation, and abrasions. It helps to improve circulatory problems such as hemorrhoids and varicose veins. The skin benefits greatly from yarrow oil as it helps with scars, stretch marks, and dry skin conditions such as eczema. Yarrow oil is also good for the scalp and helps to promote hair growth.

Properties: anti-inflammatory, antirheumatic, antiseptic, antispasmodic, astringent, carminative, cicatrisant, diaphoretic, digestive, emmenagogue, expectorant, febrifuge, stomachic, tonic, vulnerary.

Ways to Use Yarrow Essential Oil

Aging Skin – yarrow oil has a tightening effect on the muscles and skin of the face and neck, helping to improve skin sagging and tone. Mix 4 drops with 1 teaspoon of coconut oil, and massage into the face and neck.

Arthritis & Rheumatism – yarrow oil helps to improve circulation, which prevents the accumulation of uric crystals in muscles and joints. Mix 4 drops with 1 teaspoon of carrier oil, and massage into the affected area.

Chest Infections – yarrow oil helps to expel mucus from the respiratory tract and clear the infection that caused the disorder. Add 3 drops to a steam inhalation, or mix 4 drops with 1 teaspoon of carrier oil, and massage into the chest.

Constipation – yarrow oil helps to maintain a healthy digestion by regulating the secretion of digestive juices and ensuring the proper absorption of nutrients in the digestive tract, all of which result in regular bowel movements. Mix 4 drops with 1 teaspoon of carrier oil, and massage into the abdomen in a clockwise direction.

Coughing – yarrow oil has a relaxing effect on spasms within the respiratory tract, which result in persistent coughing. Mix 4 drops with 1 teaspoon of carrier oil, and massage into the chest area. You can also add 3 drops to a steam inhalation.

Cuts & Wounds – yarrow oil possesses potent antiseptic properties making it effective in treating and healing wounds at a faster rate. Mix 3 drops with 1 teaspoon of coconut oil, and massage over the area of concern twice per day.

Detox – dilute 5 drops with 1 tablespoon of carrier oil, and add to an Epsom salt bath. You can also mix 4 drops with 1 teaspoon of carrier oil, and massage into the feet. Yarrow oil promotes perspiration, which helps to speed up the removal of toxins and wastes from the body.

Eczema – yarrow oil helps to reduce inflammation of the skin, add moisture to dry skin, heal skin lesions, and prevent any infection from occurring. Mix 3 drops with 1 teaspoon of coconut oil, and massage over the area of concern.

Fever – yarrow oil is a very effective oil to use during a fever as it helps to cool the body temperature down, fight the infection that resulted in the fever, and reduce any internal inflammations that may accompany the fever. Diffuse 4 drops, or mix 4 drops with 1 teaspoon of carrier oil, and massage it into the chest area or feet.

Flatulence – yarrow oil helps to relieve pressure in the intestines by releasing gases that have built up. It is also useful in preventing the build up of gas. Mix 4 drops with 1 teaspoon of carrier oil, and massage into the abdomen in a clockwise direction.

Hair Loss – yarrow oil has excellent astringent properties and is therefore an effective treatment for preventing hair loss as it tightens hair follicles and strengthens the actual hair. Dilute 6 drops with 1 tablespoon of coconut oil, and massage into the scalp to penetrate the oils and stimulate circulation and nerve endings.

Hemorrhaging – yarrow oil contains hemostatic properties, which means it can help to contract blood vessels and stop any bleeding. Add 3 drops to a cold compress and place over the affected area.

Hemorrhoids – yarrow oil's anti-inflammatory and antiseptic properties are beneficial for treating hemorrhoids. Add 2 drops to a cold compress, and hold over the hemorrhoids for 5 minutes. You can also dilute 4 drops in 1 tablespoon of carrier oil and add to a sitz bath. Sit for 20 minutes.

High Blood Pressure – yarrow oil helps to reduce high blood pressure by having a stimulating effect on blood circulation. Mix 2 drops with ½ teaspoon of carrier oil, and massage over the heart. Repeat 2-3 times per week, followed by a week off.

Pimples & Blemishes – the powerful antiseptic, antibacterial, and anti-inflammatory properties contained within yarrow oil make it an effective treatment to help clear blemishes and prevent them from spreading. Mix 2 drops with ½ teaspoon of coconut oil, and dab over each blemish twice per day.

Scarring – yarrow oil helps to diminish the appearance of scar tissue or long term scars caused by pimples or wounds. Mix 3 drops with 1 teaspoon of coconut oil, and massage over the area twice per day.

Stomach Cramps – yarrow oil helps to relieve stomach spasms and reduce any inflammation. Mix 4 drops with 1 teaspoon of carrier oil, and massage into the abdomen in a clockwise direction.

Swollen Glands – yarrow oil helps to reduce inflamed glands, kill any infection that may be present, and increase circulation around the area. Mix 3 drops with 1 teaspoon of carrier oil and very gently massage over the area of concern, always in the direction of the heart.

Tooth Loss – the astringent properties contained within yarrow oil help to prevent tooth loss by tightening and strengthening the gums. Mix 2 drops with 1 teaspoon of aloe vera gel and massage into the gums. Leave for 5 minutes. Do not swallow. You can also create a mouth rinse by adding 2 drops to a small glass of water. Rinse mouth for 60 seconds, do not swallow.

Varicose Veins – mix 4 drops of yarrow oil with 1 tablespoon of coconut oil, and massage the affected limb in the direction of the heart. Start from the bottom of the leg and massage upwards. Very gently massage on either side of the varicose veins, never directly over them. Yarrow oil helps to stimulate and increase a slow, sluggish circulation, improving the appearance of varicose veins over time.

Ylang Ylang

Calming in times of stress, this oil helps to promote relaxation, slow a rapid heartbeat, decrease high blood pressure, and improve mood. It is a perfect oil to use for combination skin as it helps to balance sebum production for both oily and dry skin. It can also diminish the appearance of scars when applied regularly.

Properties: antidepressant, anti-inflammatory, antiseptic, antispasmodic, aphrodisiac, hypotensive, sedative.

Ways to Use Ylang Ylang Essential Oil

Acne – ylang ylang oil helps to draw out any impurities from pimples (please be aware that the pimple might get worse before it gets better as the impurities are drawn out faster but it will heal at a faster rate). Apply 1 drop of the oil directly onto the pimple using a cotton bud. Repeat twice per day.

Anger – ylang ylang oil helps to regulate the flow of adrenaline in our body and is therefore an excellent natural treatment if you need to calm down after a difficult situation. Diffuse 5 drops, or apply 3 drops on a tissue, and inhale several times an hour until you start to feel more calm and relaxed.

Anxiety – ylang ylang oil helps to calm the nervous system and is therefore a useful treatment for anyone suffering from anxiety or nervous tension. Diffuse 5 drops of ylang ylang oil, or apply 2 drops on a tissue and inhale throughout the day. Alternatively mix 6 drops of the oil with 1 tablespoon of carrier oil, and massage into the upper body. Repeat daily as and when is needed.

Aphrodisiac – diffuse 3 drops of ylang ylang, or dilute 4 drops of the oil with 1 tablespoon of carrier oil, and massage into the chest, shoulders, front and back of the neck, and the arms.

Bereavement – because ylang ylang oil has a sedative and calming effect on the body, it is a useful treatment in times of bereavement. Diffuse 5 drops of the oil, or apply 2-3 drops on a tissue and inhale throughout the day.

Dry Skin – ylang ylang oil helps to balance sebum production in the skin. Mix 4 drops of the oil with 1 teaspoon of coconut oil and massage into the skin. Leave the oil on the skin to absorb. Repeat regularly as part of your skincare routine. It can also have a positive effect on oily skin.

Emotional Upset – diffuse 5 drops of ylang ylang oil, or apply 2 drops onto a tissue and inhale throughout the day. Ylang ylang oil is a natural antidepressant and helps to instil feelings of happiness and joy.

Healthy Hair – add 5 drops to 2 ounces of shampoo to promote healthy, shiny, lustrous hair.

High Blood Pressure – ylang ylang oil helps to reduce high blood pressure. Diffuse 5 drops of the oil, or dilute 4 drops with 1 tablespoon of carrier oil and add to a bath. Soak for 20 minutes. Repeat no more than 2 times per week.

Hyperpnea (fast, shallow breathing) – diffuse 5 drops of ylang ylang oil, and allow the aroma to fill the room. Ylang ylang oil helps to slow breathing, instilling calmness to the system.

Insomnia – massaging a blend of 4 drops of ylang ylang oil with 1 teaspoon of carrier oil will help to promote a good night's sleep by relaxing the mind and body.

Muscular Spasms – dilute 5 drops of ylang ylang oil into 1 tablespoon of carrier oil and add to a warm bath. Soak for 20 minutes. Ylang ylang helps to relax muscles.

Tachycardia (over-rapid heartbeat) – mix 2 drops of ylang ylang oil with 1 teaspoon of carrier oil, massage over the heart and receive the benefit of ylang ylang's calming and sedative properties.

Worry or Fear – ylang ylang's sedative action on the autonomic nervous system will instil a sense of peace and calm to a worrying or fearful situation. Diffuse 4 drops of the oil, or apply 2 drops on a tissue and inhale regularly.

References

Patricia Davis, *Aromatherapy An A-Z*. Vermission, 2005.

Salvatore Battaglia, *The Complete Guide to Aromatherapy*. The International Centre of Holistic Therapy, 2003.

Julia Lawless, *The encyclopaedia of Essential Oils*. Element Books Limited, Great Britain, 1992.

Valerie Worwood, *The Fragrant Mind*. Doubleday, Great Britain, 1995.

Robert Tisserand, T Balacs, *Essential Oil Safety*. Churchill Livingstone, England, 1995.

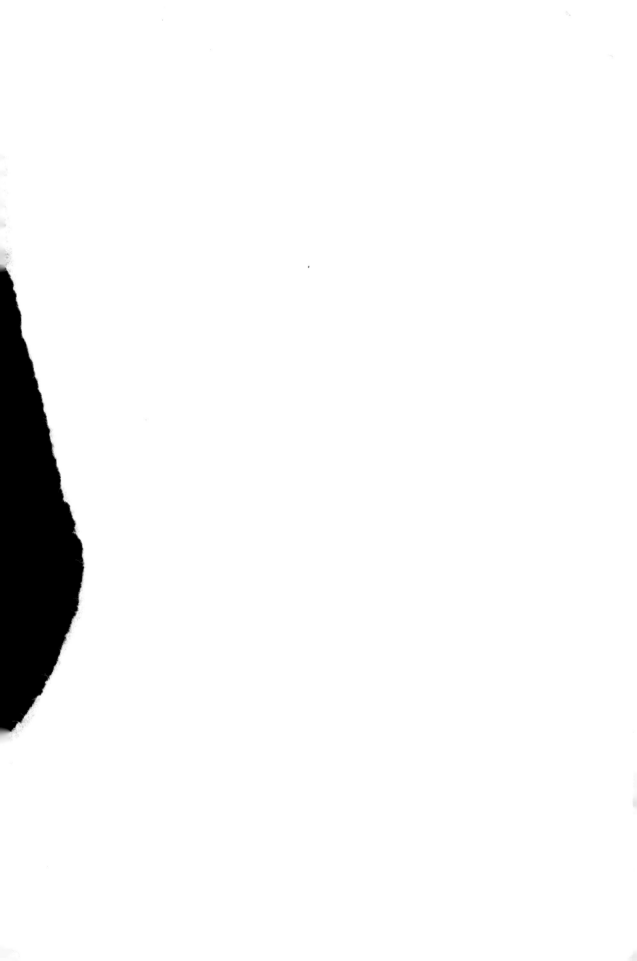

Made in the USA
Lexington, KY
09 May 2017